Thai Yoga Massage

Thai Yoga Massage

HOW TO USE TRADITIONAL THAI MASSAGE, YOGA, AND BREATHWORK FOR HEALING AND SPIRITUAL HARMONY

Thorsons

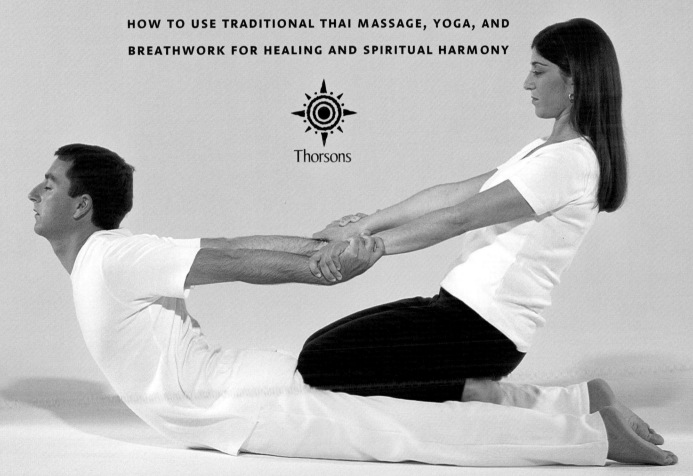

Kira Balaskas

Thorsons

An Imprint of HarperCollins*Publishers*
77–85 Fulham Palace Road
Hammersmith, London W6 8JB

The Thorsons website address is www.thorsons.com

and *Thorsons* are trademarks of
HarperCollins*Publishers* Limited

Published by Thorsons 2002

10 9 8 7 6 5 4 3 2 1

Text copyright © Kira Balaskas 2002
Copyright © HarperCollins*Publishers* Ltd 2002

Kira Balaskas asserts the moral right to be identified
as the author of this work

Designer: Liz Hallam
Photographer: Guy Hearn
Illustrations: PCA

A catalogue record for this book is available from the
British Library

ISBN 0-00-713232-8

Printed and bound in the UK by Bath Press

NOTE FROM THE PUBLISHER
This book is written to give you a flavour of Thai
yoga massage. It is in no way meant to replace good
instruction with a qualified and competent teacher.
If you are interested in learning Thai yoga massage,
whether professionally or as an effective healing art
to practise on family and friends, you will definitely
need to seek proper training. See Resources on p173
for further details.

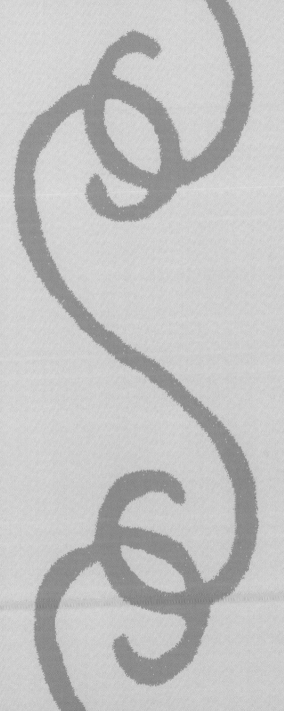

DEDICATION

To Asokananda,
It is with gratitude and appreciation that I dedicate this book to you. I would like to honour you for all the knowledge and teaching that you have shared with me. I also want to acknowledge that much of the practical information in this book has come from you and your pioneering work. I thank you for your support and encouragement during the writing of this book and for your friendship over the years.

And to my beautiful son, Alexander, who was growing inside me during the writing of this book.

ACKNOWLEDGEMENTS

My thanks go to the following people for their support during the writing of this book: my partner Mario Constantine for his help and patience, especially during the photo sessions. To my mother, Mina Semyon and step mother, Janet Balaskas for their encouragement, care and advice. To Maya Vaughan for her help and contribution. I would also like to thank John Oakley for his invaluable friendship and kindness. A big thankyou to the team at Thorsons, Belinda Budge, Nicky Vimpany and Kate Latham.

*May all misfortunes be averted, may all diseases be cured,
may no dangers be for you and may you live long and happily.*

*May all blessings be yours, may all Devas protect you. By the
power of remembering the lives of all Buddhas, their
teachings and all seekers for truth, may you always live in
safety and peace.*

From the *Mahajayamangala Gatha*

Contents

Foreword

Good books on Thai yoga massage are hard to find. Congratulations to Kira for presenting this ancient art in an authentic way. Her work shows her deep love for the practice of traditional Thai massage, a love that we have both shared for many years.

I will never forget a class I was teaching back in 1990, with a young woman enthusiastically embracing Thai yoga massage. The woman had just had a motorcycle accident and had broken one arm, but she was so keen to get started with Thai massage that nothing in the world could stop her from participating in this beginners' class, not even a serious injury, and she ended up being the most skilful student in the whole group. This young woman was Kira Balaskas and her enthusiasm for Thai yoga massage is as alive today as it was 12 years ago. Kira has been studying with me and other Thai massage teachers for many years and she is now arguably one of the foremost teachers of the tradition in the West.

In 1990 Thai massage had just started to emerge from the state of obscurity it had been pushed into by the advance of Western medicine. In the mid 80's, at the time when I became fascinated by it, Thai massage had seemed to be a dying art. Chemical drugs had replaced home remedies and traditional cures, and the reputation of Thai massage had sunk to the point of being regarded as quack practice. This was not helped by the fact that thinly disguised prostitution in massage parlors was masquerading as 'Thai massage'. Substandard massages offered at the beaches and in some commercial massage places made matters worse.

The picture changed considerably in the late 80's. The limits of Western style medicine became apparent, bringing about a massive revival of interest in alternative health care. Since the mid 90's, massage schools have begun mushrooming all over Thailand, with Chiang Mai becoming one of the major centers.

Although Thai massage has made a quantum leap, becoming popular all over the world in the last few years as a genuine yoga massage, there is still very little written material available (this is true for Western languages as well as for Thai). Some of the material that has been published in recent years seems to have been compiled by people with only a very superficial understanding of the theory and practice of this ancient art.

Kira's thoroughly researched book opens up the world of Thai yoga massage to a wider public, to anyone eager to learn about this ancient form of healing.

Asokananda
Rotorua, New Zealand
May, 2002

Introduction

I was 19 years old when I first went to Thailand. I was planning to stay for three weeks – and ended up staying for three years.

I had always been familiar with massage and yoga as both my parents were yoga teachers. Stretching and massaging were part of my childhood. So I could hardly believe my luck when I experienced Thai yoga massage for the first time. To come across something that combined yoga with massage! To me, this was heaven – lying back on a white-sand, palm-fringed beach being stretched and pummelled.

Traditionally, a Thai massage would never have been given on a beach. But that was where I was introduced to Thai massage and nowadays it is a very common place to find it being practised, especially for the benefit of the tourists.

MY QUEST BEGINS

After my beach experience in the south, I travelled up to Chiang Mai in the north of Thailand, where I came across the more serious, traditional forms of Thai massage. I preferred the northern style as it was generally longer-lasting and more thorough, using stretches I had not come across in the south. On the days following a good massage, I started to notice a feeling of renewed energy and well-being. Thai massage was seriously starting to interest me.

I finally, and reluctantly, went home to London. But on arriving home, all I was interested in was returning to Thailand as soon as possible to study Thai massage. After working in London for a while, I was soon back in Thailand wandering around Chiang Mai looking for a good school of Thai massage.

A CHANCE ENCOUNTER

I stopped for lunch at my favourite vegetarian restaurant in Chiang Mai where I was going to fill out the form for a course that was due to start in a few days' time. I was not entirely happy with the impression I had got of the school as the classes looked very big and there seemed too few teachers for the number of students, but it seemed the best of the choices on offer.

As I sat there filling out the form, a foreign man at the next table, mistaking me for an Israeli, started talking to me in Hebrew. I told him I was not Israeli but we found that we could both speak Thai and so a conversation began. He told me that he was studying Thai at the moment and that there was a German man on his course who taught Thai massage in a hill tribe village north of Chiang Mai. This sounded absolutely ideal for me as my other love in Thailand was being in the hills with the tribal people.

After lunch, I went to meet the German massage teacher, whose name was Asokananda. I immediately decided to study with him. I am very grateful that Asokananda came into my life because I found his teaching so inspiring and clear. I have never looked back. Since then, Thai yoga massage has been an extremely important, nourishing and transforming force in my life.

MY LITTLE HEALING CENTRE

When I had completed a course with Asokananda, I went on to India. While travelling around, I came across a beautiful place in the foothills of the Himalayas. I found a small room in an ashram and stayed there for six months. It was a great opportunity to practise the massage I had learned.

Every day, people would come to see me to receive treatments for various problems and ailments. My room became a little healing centre of Thai massage. During that time I gained amazing results with these people. They would return to tell me that after the treatment the pain in their abdomen had gone, or that the back pain they had suffered with for years had disappeared.

Now that I know the power of Thai massage, I would not say that these results were amazing because I would not expect anything less. Nevertheless, with such good feedback from the massage, I felt I could not ignore this effective therapy. I now feel that Thai massage chose me to be one of its vessels. From that time on, I have never stopped practising, learning and believing in Thai massage.

I would like to honour Asokananda, my first teacher, for the clear and logical way he has taught Thai massage to me and many other Westerners, without compromising the true spirit and feeling of the East. In this book and in my work I endeavour to do the same.

BEST OF BOTH WORLDS

Some people are surprised when I say that my first teacher was German, and not Thai. But Asokananda gave me such a good grounding, by applying a systematic learning structure to Thai massage, that I could then go on to study with Thai teachers and add to this strong foundation.

If I had not had that foundation I imagine it would have been far more difficult and time-consuming to learn from the Thai masters. This is not because of any lack of experience, expertise or knowledge on their part but for the simple fact that my Western mind would find it hard to learn from their Eastern way of thinking and teaching. For example, when I ask one of my Thai teachers to show me an exercise again they will often show something different. For a beginner, that can be quite confusing.

Once a person has a good basic form to their massage it is then easy to add new stretches and techniques in whatever way they are taught. Thai massage is such a rich and interesting art form. There is a never-ending number of stretches and techniques. You can keep on learning forever! Thai massage is highly rewarding for the practitioner, and not just the receiver, because giving a massage is conducive to feeling peaceful and centred and this can bring a meditative quality to your life.

A JOURNEY OF DISCOVERY

In this book I would like to take you on a journey. The journey starts by preparing your body and mind to give a massage. It then moves on to giving the massage. The journey ends with cleansing yourself and relaxing after completing the massage.

Going on this journey should be a great gift in itself. It can be a wonderfully fulfilling and inspiring experience for the giver. You can already see that Thai yoga massage is not only extremely beneficial for the person receiving the massage, but is a healing experience for both people involved.

I feel passionately about this as it has been a foundation to my life's philosophy that only by looking after, healing and caring for yourself can you then care for and help others. You have heard the saying, 'Physician heal thyself.' Thai yoga massage gives you an opportunity to start, continue and deepen that process.

How to use this book

You will get the most benefit from this book by working through it chapter by chapter, in the order in which it has been written.

CHAPTER ONE

In this chapter you will find out more about Thai yoga massage, its history, origins, the theory on which it is based and more general information about this ancient system of therapy.

CHAPTER TWO

Here you will learn simple techniques to prepare yourself for giving a Thai yoga massage. This includes yoga, breathing, visualization and chanting. You can try all of the exercises in this chapter but, at first, it is a good idea to practise just one or two. When you feel that you have understood them and have experienced the benefits, you can then move on to try the others. You may find that some of the techniques suit you better than others. Try to keep practising the ones you like best and bring them into your everyday life.

CHAPTER THREE

On these pages you will cover all the practical aspects you need to be aware of when preparing to give a massage: posture, body position, contraindications, clothing and preparing the room. Make sure you read through this chapter before beginning the massage.

CHAPTER FOUR

Here you will begin the practical application of the massage. I recommend working through this chapter in the sequence that is shown. Always read the caution before you try any exercise. It is best to try one section first, practise it a few times and then move on to the next section. Always take your time to feel at ease with one part before you move on to the next part. Slowly work through the chapter in this way until you have completed the entire massage sequence.

CHAPTER FIVE

In this chapter you will be able to try some more self-help exercises to relax and release tension after giving a massage. As in Chapter Two, it is better to master one or two of the techniques first and then move on to try the others. Once again, keep practising the ones you feel good with. Do not miss out this chapter as it ensures that you will not be left feeling tired and tense after giving a treatment.

CHAPTER SIX

The final chapter covers the basic therapy treatments used in Thai yoga massage for headache, knee pain and lower back pain. It is important that you do not try these treatments until you have mastered the massage routine in Chapter Four. In this chapter, we also look more closely at the way the energy lines run. There are charts depicting the complete energy line system used in Thai yoga massage, and a section on the use of aromatherapy oils, for your reference.

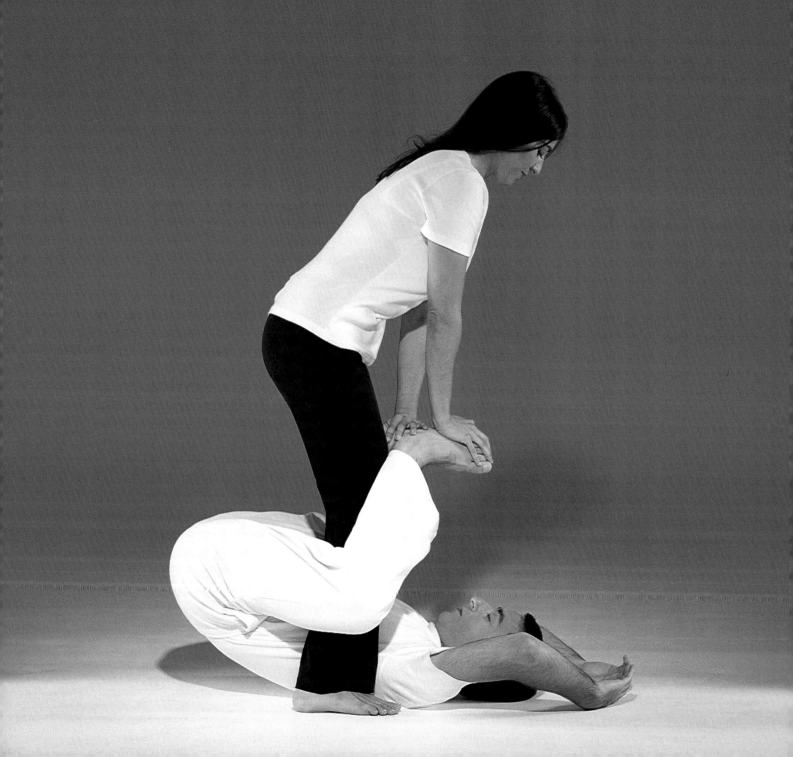

Thai Yoga Massage – Past, Present and Future

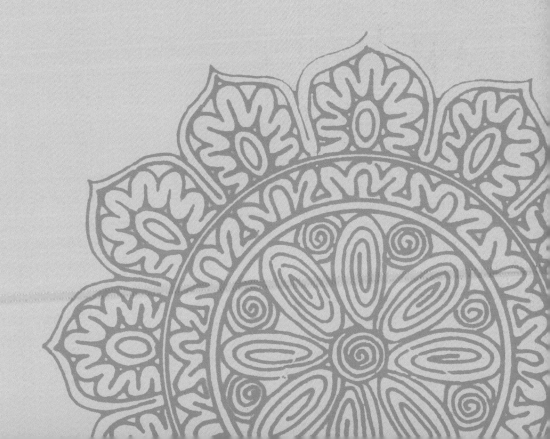

AN ANCIENT TRADITION

Thai yoga massage is a unique and powerful massage therapy, combining acupressure, gentle stretching and applied yoga. As Thai massage has grown in popularity outside Thailand, as well as inside, it has acquired a host of names. The name that I have chosen – Thai yoga massage – is just one of many that can be used to describe this ancient health system.

Whether you hear tell of 'traditional Thai massage', 'Thai yoga body-work', 'Thai traditional massage', 'nuad Thai' or 'nuad pen boran', these names all refer to the same healing art that has been practised in Thailand for thousands of years. For example, nuad pen boran is simply the phonetic translation of the Thai name for the massage system I teach. I use the name 'Thai yoga massage' because it draws attention to the yoga aspect of this method of healing.

THE ORIGINS AND HISTORY OF THAI YOGA MASSAGE

Perhaps surprisingly, the roots of Thai yoga massage are not to be found in Thailand but in northern India. The founder of this form of massage is believed to be a man called Jivaka Kumar Bhaccha, who was physician to the Maghada king Bimbisara more than 2,500 years ago, around the time that Buddha was alive.

Evidence of the existence of Jivaka Kumar Bhaccha can be found in the Theravada Buddhist scriptures, in a section called the Pali Cannon. Bhaccha, who Thai people call Shivagokumarpaj, was said to have been a close friend of Buddha. Even today, Bhaccha is honoured in Thailand as

RIGHT A Thai Buddha at the old capital of Thailand, Ayutthaya

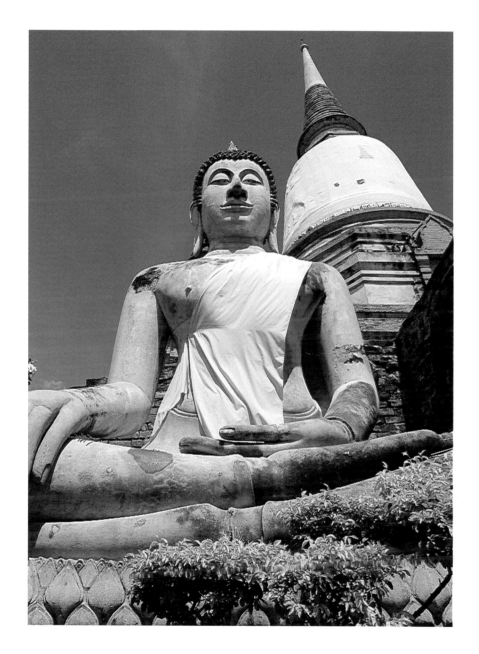

the 'father of medicine' and most schools and practitioners of Thai yoga massage say prayers each day to remember him as the founder and source of the healing art that they are practising.

It is not clear exactly how, when and in what form Thai yoga massage reached Thailand. It seems that it may have arrived in Thailand along with Buddhism around the third or second century BC. The origins of Thai yoga massage almost certainly lie in the traditional Indian system of healing. There are similarities too between aspects of Thai yoga massage and the energy pathways, or meridians, that feature in Chinese acupressure and acupuncture, and in the Japanese therapy shiatsu.

So much of the history of Thai yoga massage is unknown that we can only hazard a guess as to whether there was ever an indigenous form of massage in Thailand and, if so, to what extent it was influenced by Chinese medicine.

However, any similarities are only superficial as the Thai system of *sen* lines differs markedly from the network of energy pathways described in these other healing traditions.

There are various reasons why the origins of Thai yoga massage have remained obscure. It is partly due to the fact that for centuries Thai medical knowledge was mostly passed down orally from teacher to pupil rather than written down. Another reason is that much of the early written records have been lost. Some Thai medical scriptures were set down on palm leaves, in the ancient language Pali. This language is similar to that spoken in northern India at the time of the Buddha. Most of the medical scriptures were destroyed in 1767 when Burmese invaders attacked the old capital of Thailand, Ayutthaya. However, some remnants survived and the text they contained can still be seen carved on the walls at Wat Pho (Phra Chetupon), a famous temple in Bangkok.

THAI YOGA MASSAGE TODAY

There has been a revival of Thai yoga massage in Thailand in recent years. Prior to this, the increasing popularity and accessibility of orthodox Western medicine meant that the authentic Thai forms of healing and massage were being replaced – although by no means lost. In the country villages, the traditional teachings were kept alive by masters continuing in the ancient ways of their forefathers. In Thailand's main cities, massage schools, such as Wat Pho in Bangkok and the Foundation of Shivagokumarpaj in Chiang Mai, have been working hard also to keep these healing traditions alive.

An interest in alternative forms of medicine, which developed in the West during the 1980s, brought many Westerners to Thailand in search of traditional Eastern methods of healing. This led to a resurgence of interest in Thai yoga massage. Since then it has become increasingly popular, both in Thailand and in the West.

The people and government of Thailand now recognise that Thai yoga massage is far superior to conventional Western medicine in the treatment of many ailments. For example, it can often be more effective than physiotherapy or medication in helping people to recover after a stroke, by returning mobility and feeling to their limbs. It is also extremely effective in treating frozen shoulder, asthma, back pain and many other conditions.

Nowadays, you will find many massage schools in Chiang Mai offering courses in Thai yoga massage. And there are establishments offering massage treatments on almost every street corner. However, because of commercial exploitation of Thai yoga massage, the quality of training and treatment is not always of the highest standard.

In other parts of the world, the number of schools of Thai yoga massage is on the increase and so there are now more and more people practising this form of healing. As Thai yoga massage is still relatively new to most countries, their governments have not yet brought in regulations covering the standard of massage. As a consequence, the quality of some of the treatments and of the training on offer can be quite low. The problem being that the masseurs and teachers themselves often lack adequate training and experience.

However, things are improving all the time and I am sure it will not be long before Thai yoga massage becomes more tightly regulated around the world. There are many dedicated and experienced Thai masseurs and teachers currently setting more stringent standards for Thai yoga massage. I am involved in this process in England, Asokananda (see Resources on page 173) is doing the same in New Zealand, and there are others I know of working in Germany, Italy and Austria. So, if you are looking for professional training or treatment, I suggest you seek out someone who teaches or practises in the true spirit of this beautiful healing art.

THAI YOGA MASSAGE STYLES

There are two general styles of Thai yoga massage practised in Thailand – northern and southern. The principal school for southern style is at Wat Pho, in Bangkok. The main centre for the northern style is at the Old Medicine Hospital of the Foundation of Shivagokumarpaj, in Chiang Mai. However, there has recently been an upsurge in the number of schools teaching Thai yoga massage in Chiang Mai and you can now find them all over the city.

Southern-style Thai massage tends to be shorter than the northern form. Sessions last one hour only and do not include as many stretches as

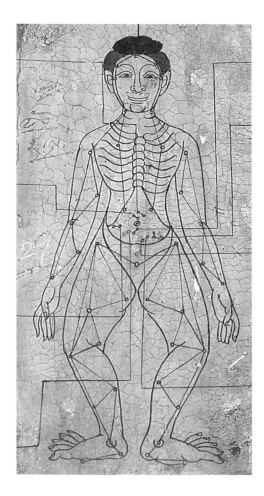

An ancient epigraph at Wat Pho
(Phra Chetupon), Bangkok

the other approach. Northern-style Thai massage, on the other hand, usually lasts for two to two-and-a-half hours and includes many yoga based stretching movements and thorough work on the energy lines of the legs.

The approach of this book is much closer to the northern style, as my own background is in this system of Thai massage. I first studied in northern Thailand with Asokananda, before going on to spend a lot of time studying with other northern Thai masters.

Even within the northern or southern approaches, you will find that there is plenty of diversity, and some people use a mixture of both styles. In fact, as you travel from place to place in Thailand, you will rarely receive the same form of treatment twice. Some practitioners mostly concentrate on energy lines, working in a very slow and thorough manner. Others include lots of stretching or tendon plucking. The length of the massage may also vary. Some schools even use hot herbal compresses at every session. I have had massages in which a hot compress was kept under my neck throughout the treatment.

Whether you receive a northern- or southern-style massage in Thailand, the quality of the massage will vary greatly. In most massage establishments, it is pot luck whether you get an experienced masseur or someone who has had three days' training and is more interested in chatting to a friend than massaging you.

The only way to guarantee a good massage is to go by personal recommendation or to seek out a master. Most true masters have probably been chosen at a very young age to study with the healer of the village, often an older relative. These people would therefore have received very skilled, in-depth training and would have been practising for many years.

THE THEORY BEHIND THAI YOGA MASSAGE

Thai yoga massage is based on a belief in a life force that circulates around special pathways in the body. Indian yoga philosophy calls this life force *prana*. It is said to be absorbed into the body from the food we eat and the air we breathe. In Thai yoga massage, these *prana* pathways make up an energy line system called *ten sen*. This system is said to be made up of 72,000 invisible energy lines called *pranamaya kosha* or the 'energy body'. If there is a blockage in any line preventing the free flow of *prana* it can lead to aches, pain and disease on a physical, emotional and spiritual level.

Thai yoga massage concentrates on 10 important lines, called *sip sen* or *ten sen*. A thorough Thai massage treatment should cover all 10 lines. By working these lines it is possible to treat the whole body, including the internal organs. This will ensure that blocked energy is released, restoring health, harmony and balance. When the *prana* is flowing freely your general well-being is greatly improved.

The Indian origins of Thai yoga massage are clear from this basic theory. The link becomes even more obvious if we compare the names of three of these main Thai yoga massage energy lines with their Indian equivalents, known as *prana nadis*. For example, the Thai energy line called *sen sumana* is known to Indian yogis as *sushumna nadi*. Similarly, *sen ittha* in Thai medicine is known as *ida nadi* to practitioners of the Indian *prana* system and *sen pingkhala* is equivaent to *pingkala nadi*.

Some people think that Thai *sen* lines are the same as the meridians featured in therapies such as Japanese shiatsu. However, this is definitely not the case as the *sen* lines follow different pathways from those of the meridians. The fact is that all these traditions work very differently. Thai yoga massage places the emphasis on working lines, whereas shiatsu emphasizes working points. This may be the original reason for using a different line system in Thai yoga massage. This line system may fulfil the purpose for Thai yoga massage better than another.

SPIRITUAL ASPECTS OF THAI YOGA MASSAGE

It is important to understand the spiritual nature of Thai yoga massage. Thai yoga massage was traditionally practised in Buddhist temples and was an extension of Buddhist practice – particularly meditation. The meditative aspects of Thai yoga massage takes two forms. Firstly, when you give a massage you should experience a sense of awareness and of being present in each moment as you work through each part of the receiver's body. Secondly, Thai yoga massage features a practice known as *metta* or 'loving kindness' meditation. Thai yoga massage is said to be 'the physical application of loving kindness'. I think that is such a beautiful description of it.

Perhaps the most important aspect of Thai yoga massage is the intention with which you give the massage. A massage given with awareness and care will feel totally different from one given in a mechanical or technical way. Giving a massage in a meditative mood is most effective for tuning into the needs of the receiver and developing your intuition for the energy flow. It will also leave you feeling calm and peaceful.

UNDERSTANDING THE DIFFERENCES BETWEEN EAST AND WEST

If we want to tune into the essence of Thai massage, or any other Asian healing tradition, we need to begin by understanding Asian thought. Without this understanding we automatically try to fit Thai massage into our Western way of seeing things. A systematic and analytical viewpoint makes it very difficult to understand Thai yoga massage, as Thai massage comes from a much more intuitive and poetic Eastern approach.

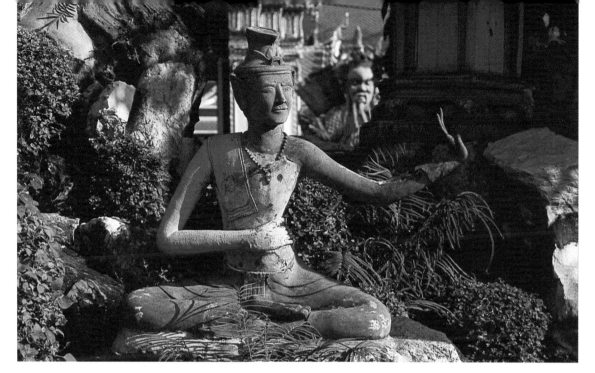
A Thai yoga massage sculpture at Wat Pho, Bangkok

In the West, we try to find one truth, one solution and one answer to things. In the East they see many ways to deal with matters and look for what feels like the right thing to do at that moment. The Eastern mind does not search for final answers but instead looks for something that will fulfil the purpose. This makes it difficult to standardize treatments and therapies in Thai massage. As there is no fixed or standard solution to a specific problem, one needs to be intuitive and creative in trying a treatment and, if it does not work, willing to try something else.

For example, in the Western medical approach, nearly everyone who goes to a doctor suffering from a stomach ulcer will be given the same treatment. With Eastern medicine, if several people went to a practitioner of Chinese medicine, each would almost certainly receive totally different treatments. The same holds true for Thai massage.

Another difference between the two approaches is that, unlike Western medicine, Thai massage has little or no understanding of Western anatomy and physiology. In ancient Thai society, the dissection of dead bodies was not permitted. Therefore, healers learned nothing of the basic structure of the body under the skin or of the physiological processes involved. Instead, Eastern medical practitioners discovered how the energy body worked and how massage could be used to heal people by releasing blockages in the energy flow.

When teaching in the West, I am aware that many people want to apply their knowledge of anatomy and physiology to Thai massage. Although there is no harm in this, I do want to make it clear that this knowledge will not improve the effectiveness and quality of the massage they give. It is important that this scientific approach does not interfere with your innate ability to sense and feel the energy flow, which is intrinsic to Thai yoga massage, and to apply Thai massage in an intuitive and creative way.

This is a wonderful aspect of Thai yoga massage: it allows you to develop this intuition and inspires a certain level of mindfulness and centredness in the giver. Intuition is a vital part of healing in the framework of Thai massage.

EFFECTS AND BENEFITS OF THAI YOGA MASSAGE

There are many benefits to be gained from a Thai massage. Practitioners are mainly concerned with balancing the energy systems of the body and therefore Thai yoga massage can have profound effects on the receiver After receiving a massage, it usually takes four or five days for this energy re-balancing to be complete. This means that people often continue to experience the beneficial effects for some time after the massage, and not just during the treatment.

There are several reactions that you can expect after receiving a massage. The two most common initial feelings are extreme tiredness, which is a sign that old and negative energy is leaving the body, and a feeling of having lots of energy, which indicates that new energy is flowing into the body.

Whatever your first reaction, you can expect that your energy will be balanced after a few days. This means that even if you felt very tired immediately afterwards, once this feeling passes you will usually be conscious of having much more energy.

Other benefits include greater flexibility in the joints, enhanced blood circulation, better alignment of the body, improved posture and additional stimulation of the internal organs, which helps them to function optimally. Thai yoga massage also gives the receiver a feeling of relaxation and tranquillity that is invaluable for today's stressful lifestyle.

WHERE TO GET PERSONAL TUITION

This book is written to give you a flavour of Thai yoga massage. In no way is it meant to replace good instruction from a qualified and competent teacher. If you are interested in learning Thai yoga massage, whether to take up a professional career as a practitioner or simply to learn an effective healing art that you can practise on family and friends, you will definitely need proper training. For more details, see the Resources at the back of this book (page 173)

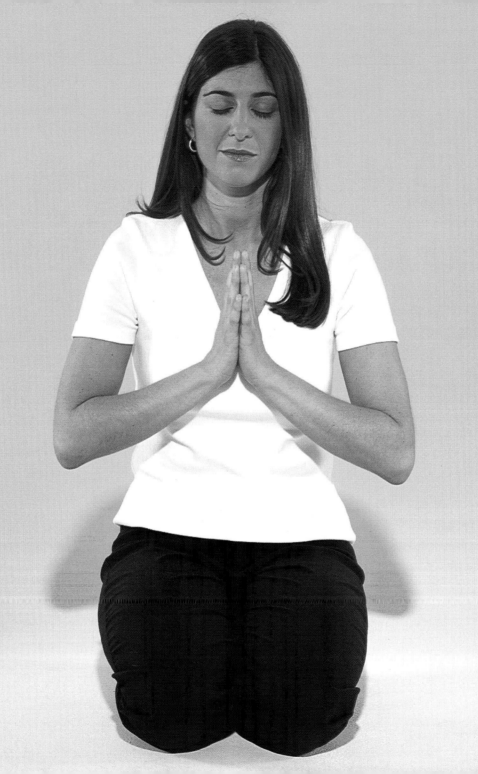

2

Self-preparation

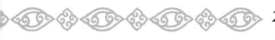

HOW TO PROTECT YOURSELF

Before you begin the massage, you should make sure that you are centred, relaxed and clear in your intention. You also need to protect yourself from any negative energy or tension that the receiver may release during the treatment. The best way to do this is with thorough self-preparation. Otherwise, giving a Thai yoga massage may well leave you feeling tense, tired and even sick. There are many methods you can use to prepare yourself, such as yoga, chi gung, t'ai chi or another discipline, either singly or in combination. The most important thing is that you find a way that works for you and suits you personally. In Thailand, most masters of Thai massage practise Theravada Buddhist meditation as their way of preparing themselves before beginning the massage and working with energy lines. In this chapter, I have included several exercises and techniques that over the years I have found useful for preparation. The techniques come from various disciplines, such as yoga and t'ai chi, and not all are traditional to Thailand.

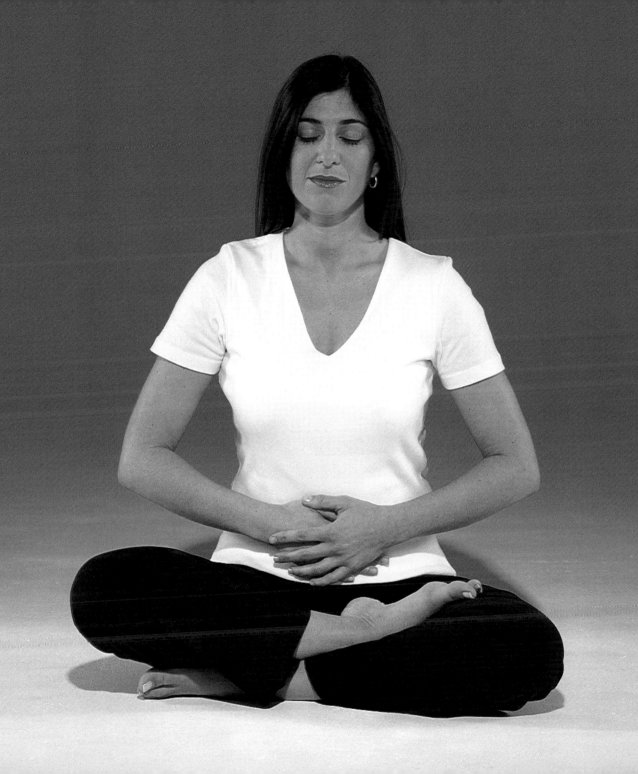

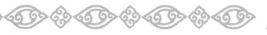

Meditation

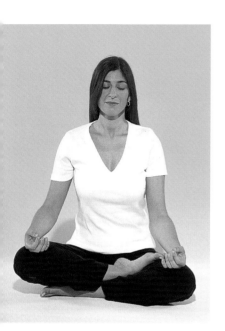

A busy mind is not conducive to giving a good massage. Meditation is an effective way of slowing down your thoughts and quietening your mind. I believe that the practice of mindfulness and meditation can benefit everybody, no matter what their beliefs or religion. There are many Buddhist schools, each one offering its own unique style of meditation. If Buddhist meditation interests you, I recommend that you find a good teacher to study the practice in more depth. In this section I would simply like to give you a few meditation exercises that you can easily use as a preparation for giving a massage.

CHOOSING A POSITION

Finding a comfortable sitting position is of great importance. The ideal position for meditation is known as the full lotus. Here, you sit with back straight and one foot (left or right) on top of the opposite thigh, tight up to the groin. The heel of the other foot rests high up on its opposite thigh. It is a very stable position and allows for optimum balance of the spine. Unfortunately, most of us are not supple enough to do the full-lotus position. Therefore you need to find a comfortable way of your own to sit, depending on your body shape and level of flexibility.

A simpler position is the half lotus. Sitting with your back straight, you bend your left (or right) knee and rest the heel of your left (or right) foot near to your body. Now bend your right (or left) knee as you lift the right (or left) foot and rest it in your groin.

Other options include kneeling, sitting cross-legged, sitting with your back against a wall or simply sitting on a chair. You could also lie on your back with your knees comfortably bent. Whichever position you choose, make sure you will be able to stay in that position for at least 10 minutes. It is advisable to choose just one of the following exercises and practise it for a month or so. Trying to do all of them at once may be too much.

MINDFULNESS PRACTICE – COUNTING THE BREATH

This is an easy technique to use to help you concentrate. In this exercise you simply count your in-breaths and out-breaths in cycles of 10. This is an exercise in concentration, observing intrusive thoughts and coming back to the breath.

Sit comfortably and close your eyes. As you inhale, be mindful that 'I am inhaling, one'. As you exhale be mindful that 'I am exhaling, one'. Continue in this way, counting each inhalation and exhalation up to 10, then start again at one.

You can repeat this as many times as you like. Whenever your mind starts to wander off, simply return to one and start again.

TOGLEN – LOVING KINDNESS MEDITATION

This exercise comes from a Tibetan practice called *toglen*. The principle behind this form of meditation is to first acknowledge the state of the world, the hatred, conflict and disharmony that is also within us. You then transform it into a higher potential of being and existence where love, peace and unity can prevail.

To start, close your eyes and take a few normal, quiet breaths. Now, as you breathe in, imagine that you are taking in all the pain, suffering and ignorance of the world. As you breathe out, imagine that compassion, wisdom, acceptance and loving kindness are flowing out of you. Repeat this cycle as many times as you wish.

FLOWER MEDITATION

A few years ago, I spent one summer in France at a place called Plum Village. This is where a Vietnamese monk named Thich Nhat Hanh has set up a monastery and retreat centre. While I was there, I learnt this lovely meditation. I recommend you try it. Start by sitting comfortably, then close your eyes and bring your attention on to your breath. Focus your attention on your breath, and the rise and fall of your abdomen, as you breathe in and out.

As you inhale, consciously think 'I am a flower'. As you exhale, think 'I feel fresh'. Repeat 20 times. Now shorten the thought on the in-breath to 'flower' and on the out-breath to 'fresh'. Repeat 20 times.

As you inhale, think 'I am a mountain' and, as you exhale, think 'I feel still'. Repeat 20 times. Now shorten the thought on the in-breath to 'mountain' and on the out-breath to 'still'. Repeat 20 times.

As you inhale, think 'I am water' and, as you exhale, think 'I am reflecting'. Repeat 20 times. Now shorten the thought on the in-breath to 'water' and on the out-breath to 'reflecting'. Repeat 20 times.

As you inhale, think 'I am space' and, as you exhale, think 'I feel free'. Repeat 20 times. Now shorten the thought on the in-breath to 'space' and on the out-breath to 'free'. Repeat 20 times.

RIGHT A statue of a meditating Buddha at Wat Arun, Bangkok

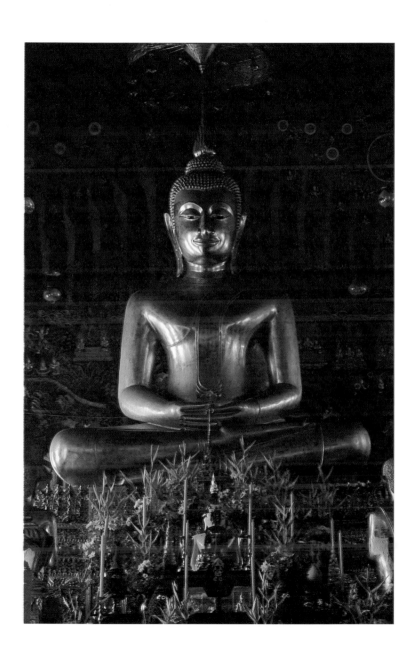

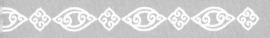

Breathing exercises

Breathing well is the key to being truly relaxed. You may notice that when you feel nervous or stressed you experience a shortness of breath and your rate of breathing increases. By breathing more deeply and slowing your breath down you exert a positive influence on your general state of being, physically, mentally and emotionally.

Sit comfortably, as in the previous meditations. Close your eyes and become aware of your breath. Gently focus your attention on the rise and fall of your abdomen as you inhale and exhale. When your breathing feels comfortable, you can begin.

NADI SODHANA – ALTERNATE NOSTRIL BREATHING

This is a yoga practice that helps to improve the flow of your breath through the nasal passages. It is also a powerful way to balance the energy flow and energize the Prana body. Place the thumb of your left hand gently on your left nostril. Place your ring and little finger gently on your right nostril, allowing your index and middle finger to curl naturally inside your hand. Ensure that your touch is very light to avoid straining your neck.

Close your left nostril with your thumb. Now breathe in through your right nostril for a count of four. Close your right nostril with your ring and little finger, release your thumb and breathe out of your left nostril for a count of four. Now breathe in through the left nostril, close with your thumb, release the ring and little finger and breathe out through the right nostril. Repeat this cycle 10 times, then relax and breathe normally for 10 breaths.

KUMBAKA – BREATH RETENTION EXERCISE

This is a another yoga exercise that helps expand the lung capacity, allowing you to breathe more fully. Breathe in for a count of four. Pause and hold the breath for a count of 12. Breathe out for a count of eight. Pause for a moment and then allow the in-breath to happen naturally. Repeat this cycle 10 times. Now relax and take 10 normal breaths.

Try to relax into the pause, taking care not to tense up as you hold the breath for a count of 12. If you feel any strain it is better to hold for a shorter time, as long as you keep to the ratio of one:three:two. For example, you could breathe in for a count of two, hold for a count of six and breathe out for a count of four.

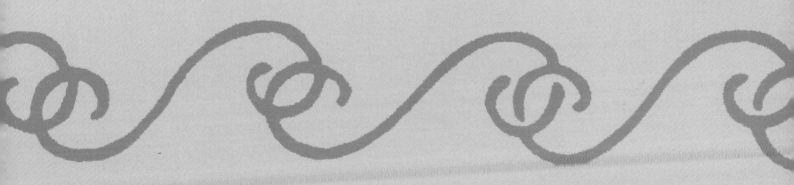

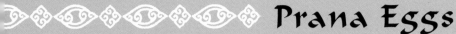
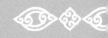

Prana Eggs

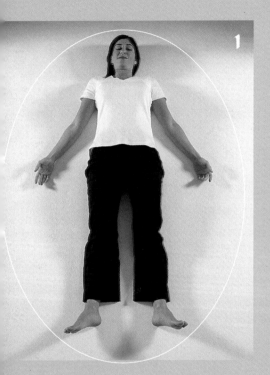

Visualization is a powerful technique that can be used on its own or, as here, combined with breathing to still troubled thoughts and aid relaxation. The following visualizations are called *prana* eggs because they are made up of your breath – and, hence, your life force *prana* – which you use to form an egg shape in your mind. They offer an excellent way to protect your energy field and ward off negative energies that may have been released by the receiver.

Prana Eggs is in three parts. The first part protects you from external energy influences. The second part helps you to develop self-confidence and gives you a feeling of balance and calm. The third part induces a state of deep rest and relaxation.

To start, lie comfortably on your back with your head pointing north. This makes best use of the Earth's polarity. Keep your arms relaxed by your sides, palms facing up. Allow your legs to rest evenly on the floor.

Take a deep in-breath. As you do so, imagine you are drawing a line in a half-oval shape, starting about 10 cm (4 in) below your toes and coming up on the right side of your body until it reaches about 10 cm (4 in) above your head.

Now breathe out, and as you do so imagine drawing the other half of the oval, starting at the same point above your head, coming down the left side of your body and finishing at the same point below your toes. You are now lying in the centre of a big egg shape. Repeat this nine times.

2 As you breathe in, again draw a line in a half-oval shape, but this time starting at the toes (not below them), running along the right side of your body and ending at your head (not above it). Now breathe out, continuing the other half of the oval down the left side of the body, finishing at your toes again. Repeat nine times.

3 Again, begin by breathing in, but this time imagine beginning the line at the pelvis. Follow the line up in a half oval on the right side and stop at the point between your eyebrows. As you breathe out, continue the oval on the left side and finish at the pelvis. Repeat nine times.

In many Eastern beliefs, the body is said to have seven energy centres, or chakras. The pelvis contains the base chakra, and the point between the eyebrows is known as the third-eye chakra.

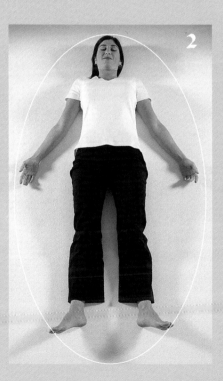

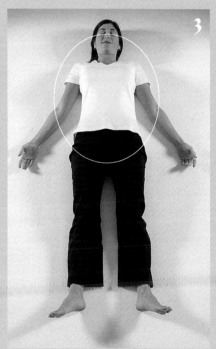

 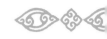

Centring

When giving a Thai yoga massage, it is important to be open, relaxed and centred. This allows the universal, or cosmic, energy to flow into your body and replenish the energy that you are giving out. If you can find a place of balance and centredness inside yourself, you are in an ideal state to give a massage.

Giving a massage is a powerful way of seeing your relationship to giving and is a wonderful way of bringing this relationship into balance. As a first step, it is essential to find a place of balance within yourself as this helps you to avoid absorbing the receiver's negative energy and prevents you from feeling drained and tired afterwards. It also stops any negative or tense energy in you from flowing into the receiver. The following exercise helps you find that place of centredness within.

MAKING CONTACT WITH YOUR CENTRE OF GRAVITY

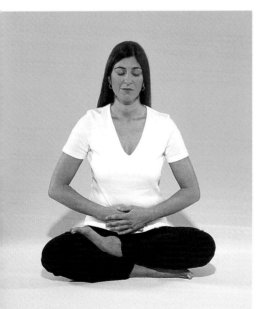

Start by sitting cross-legged or kneeling. Place your hands just below your navel. Close your eyes and take 10 deep breaths, focusing your mind on the rising of the abdomen as you breathe in and the falling of the abdomen as you breathe out. Give yourself a few moments to feel the rising and falling of your abdomen underneath your hands. This area is your centre of gravity or *hara*.

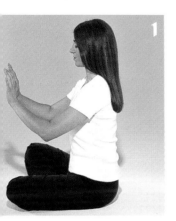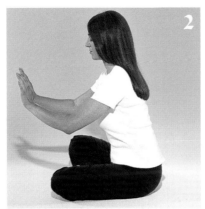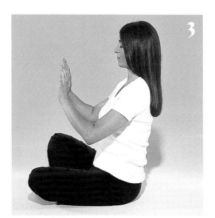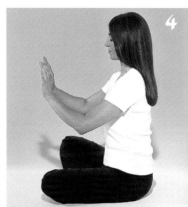

1 Now hold your hands out in front of you with your palms facing away from you and your arms slightly bent.

2 Keeping your shoulders relaxed and your breathing steady, begin to straighten your arms by gently pushing your palms forwards until you sense that you are losing your awareness of your centre of gravity. You will feel slightly off balance as if you are falling forwards. Now come back to your original position.

3 Try bending your elbows and slowly bring your hands back towards your body, still with your palms facing forwards, until you begin to feel off balance again, as if falling backwards. Now slowly bring yourself back.

4 Push your hands forwards again, this time only reaching as far as you can without losing your centre of gravity. Find the place of perfect balance within yourself for giving. This is where you can most comfortably give. Take a few minutes to really feel that place. Remember this feeling so that you can remind yourself of it when giving the massage.

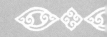

Simple Yoga Positions

You are often required to kneel when giving Thai yoga massage. So you will need to have a few comfortable positions to choose from so that you can easily change from one to another when one position becomes tiring. These positions require a certain amount of flexibility in the hips and ankles.

Do not worry if you are not already flexible because as you practise you will see a noticeable improvement. That is the beauty of Thai yoga massage, it will inspire you to become more flexible and free in your body, which in turn enhances your well-being and improves your life in general. The following exercises will improve your flexibility before you begin working on the floor.

LOOSENING UP ANKLES – THREE-WAY ANKLE STRETCH

Sit on your heels with your feet as close together as possible. Relax your weight down on to your heels and take 10 deep breaths. If this is too painful for you, place a cushion on top of your legs and under your buttocks so that you are raised slightly, sitting on the cushion.

This first position stretches and opens the ankles.

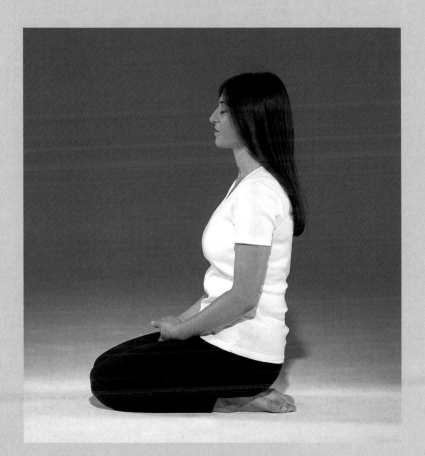

Come up on to your knees and then turn your toes under. Now sit back on to your heels again and gently and slowly release your weight down. Take 10 deep breaths. If your toes start to hurt, come forwards and put the weight on your hands. Then sit back again for only as many breaths as feels bearable. This second position stretches the ankles in a different direction, adds a stretch to the toes and stimulates some therapeutic points on the feet.

This stretches the ankles and toes, and stimulates therapy points.

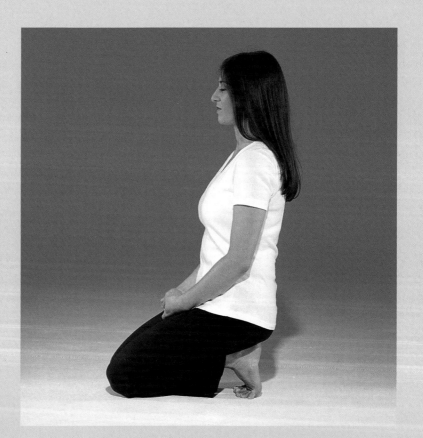

Now bring your knees off the floor and sit back in a squatting position, taking your heels as close to the floor as possible. Open your knees and allow your body to fold forwards in front of you between your knees. Take 10 deep breaths each time, dropping your heels lower to the floor. If you cannot get your heels anywhere near the floor, place the edge of a cushion under them. This position stretches the ankles in a third direction and helps to open the hips.

Now come back into the second position, pause for a few breaths, then come back into first position, sitting on your heels again. You should feel more comfortable than when you started.

This position stretches the ankles and opens the hips.

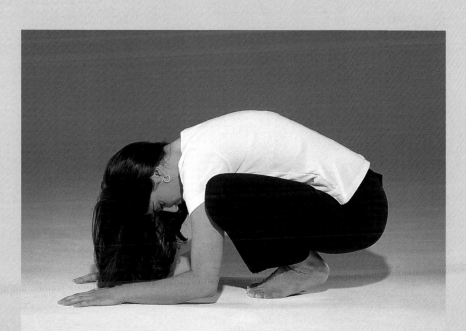

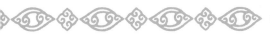 # Chanting

This is a powerful way to clear the mind and can quickly and effectively induce a feeling of inner peace. Chanting has a wonderfully soothing effect and is ideal as a preparation for giving Thai yoga massage. Many traditions and religions use chanting in their ceremonies or rituals. I have mainly come across Hindu and Tibetan chants in India, and Pali chants in Thailand. The ancient language Pali is now used mainly for chanting in Theravada Buddhism.

While I was travelling in Dharamsala, the place where the majority of Tibetans who moved to northern India came to settle, I was lucky enough to witness an amazing ceremony. The Dalai Lama was giving a talk at two in the morning, during full moon, for the celebration of the Buddha's birthday. I was outside, under the moon, with 5,000 Tibetans – and the atmosphere was incredible. After a while, I realised that they were all repeating certain words over and over again.

These words were *Om Mani Padme Hum*. Later on, when I went to study Thai yoga massage with Asokananda, I found that he started each class by chanting this mantra. I have continued this tradition in my classes and also when by myself as a preparation for the day.

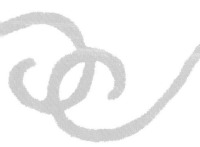

Om Mani Padme Hum is a powerful mantra of understanding and compassion. Much has been written on the meaning of this mantra. Here, I give you an extremely simplified translation:

Om is the sound or vibration
of the universe.

Mani is a jewel or a diamond
that is a symbol of beauty and light
and has the sharpness to cut through ignorance.

Padme is a lotus flower symbolizing beauty
that can rise up out of the mud and blossom.
The mud is our ignorance and the lotus
is compassion and wisdom.

Hum means to bring together, to unify.

When combined, the words mean:

The lotus flower is growing out of the mud.
The jewel in the centre of the lotus flower
shines forth the light of love and compassion,
which unites with the sound of the universe
creating cosmic harmony.

Another chant that I learned from Asokananda is in Pali and is taken from a chant called 'the great peaceful victory'. It is a beautiful blessing.

In the Pali language:

Sabbitiyo vivajantu-sabbarogo vinasatu
ma te bhavato anterayo-sukhi dighayuko bhave

Bhavatu sabbamangalam-rakkhantu sabbadevata
sabbabuddhanubhavena-sada sotthi bhanantu te

Bhanatu sabbamangalam-rakkantu sabbadevata
sabbadhamannubhavena-sada sotthi bhavantu te

Bhavatu sabbamangalam-rakantu sabbadevata
Sabbasanghannubhavena-sada sotthi bhavatu te.

In English:

> May all misfortunes be averted, may all diseases be cured,
> may no dangers be for you and may you live long and happily.
>
> May all blessings be yours, may all Devas protect you.
> By the power of remembering the lives of all Buddhas,
> their teachings and all seekers for truth,
> may you always live in safety and peace.

What a lovely thing to wish for the receiver as you give them a massage!

Although it is impossible to learn the tunes for these chants from a book, you can be creative and come up with your own way of chanting the words.

I recommend Asokananda's book *Thus Have I Heard*. It includes many chants and their translations that go with a CD or audio cassette tape (*see Resources on page 173*).

Another option is to find a teacher who can show you how. There are so many beautiful chants, it is certainly worth the effort.

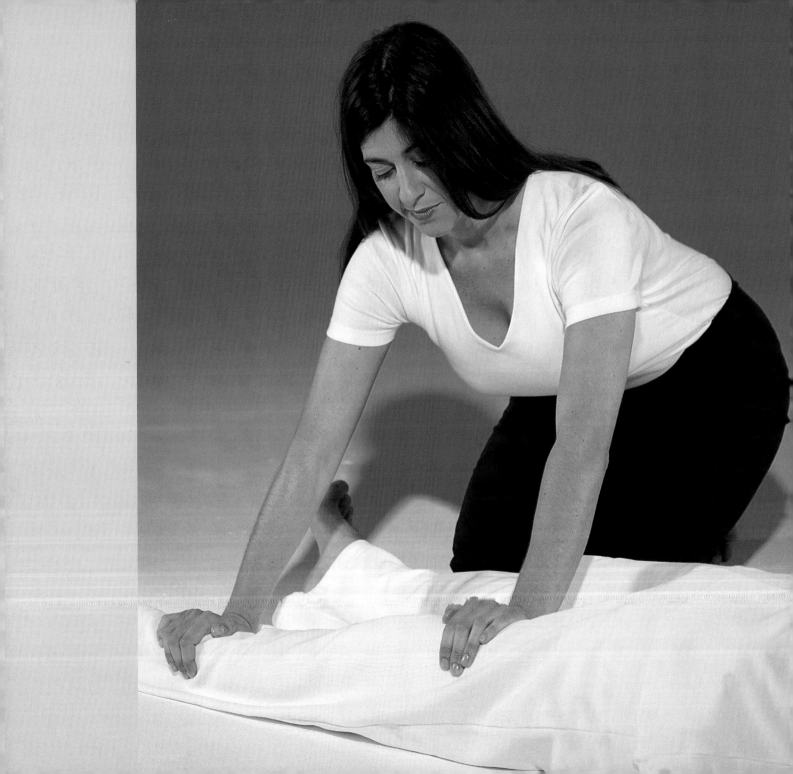

3

Practical
Considerations

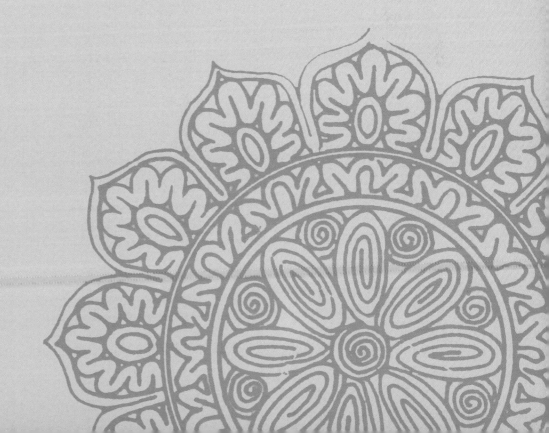

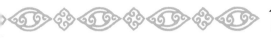 

Be Prepared

To give Thai yoga massage you will need enough room for a mat and plenty of space to move all around it. It is more harmonious to receive a massage in an uncluttered space so the clearer the room the better. The receiver should lie on a mat that is neither too thick nor too soft. A thin futon is ideal. If you do not have a mat, two simple alternatives are to use a few folded blankets or a duvet.

The room should be a comfortable temperature for both you and the receiver. Lying still for a long time can lower the body temperature, so it is important that the receiver does not get too cold. But at the same time you, as the giver, will be moving around a great deal and if the room is very warm you may well get too hot. I have found the best way to overcome this problem is to keep towels or blankets warming on a radiator. I use these to cover my client. This enables you to keep the receiver warm without getting too hot yourself. In Thailand, warm towels are totally unnecessary, owing to the warm climate. But in England, where I have been working, they go down a treat with my clients.

CREATING THE RIGHT AMBIENCE

If you like, you can burn incense or aromatherapy oils to make the room smell nice. If you need lighting, make sure it is not too bright and position the light so that it is not shining in the receiver's eyes. Lighted candles offer an easy way to create a peaceful atmosphere.

The room should be as kept quiet as possible. Choose a time when you are not expecting visitors and unplug or switch off the telephone so you will not be disturbed.

CHECK THE HEALTH OF YOUR PATIENT

Before you begin the massage you MUST ask the receiver about their health. This is because it is essential to know about any condition that would make massage unsafe or inadvisable, to avoid causing harm in any way. In medical terminology, a reason for avoiding giving a particular treatment is known as a 'contraindication'.

In Thailand, it is not usual practice to ask the receiver to fill out a health questionnaire. However, the practice is mandatory in the West and is taught in all bodywork training.

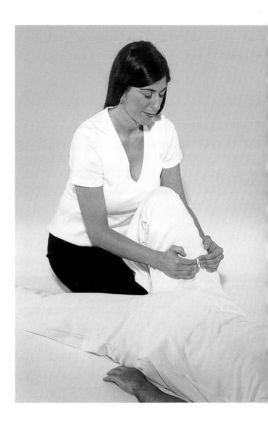

The most important thing is that you are aware of the information. If you are practising Thai yoga massage professionally, it is essential to use a health questionnaire so that you have a permanent record of the information. But when planning a private massage to be performed on a partner, friend or member of the family it is sufficient just to ask the person verbally.

Here is an example of a typical questionnaire. In addition to their name, address and telephone number, you will need to include questions such as the following:

- Do you have low or high blood pressure?
- Do you have a heart problem?
- Do you have varicose veins?
- Have you had any recent operations?
- Do you have any skin diseases?
- Do you wear contact lenses?
- Are you pregnant?
- Are you menstruating?

⊛ Do you have any stomach or intestinal problems?
⊛ Is there any part of your body that is tender, achy or especially sensitive?
⊛ Do you suffer from any other medical problems or health conditions?

PREGNANCY

If you are a beginner, it is not advisable to practise massage on a pregnant woman until you have gained plenty of experience and confidence. Thai yoga massage is wonderful in pregnancy. An experienced practitioner will have plenty of techniques to apply a good, full body massage to a pregnant woman. This can be applied while the woman is lying on her side.

Although many of the techniques and exercises in this book can be safely applied in pregnancy, a full body massage would not be possible, as not all the techniques needed for this are covered here. There is a form of abdominal massage involving a very light touch that can be used in pregnancy, but it is not included in this introductory book.

So, as you will not be learning this special form, do not massage the abdomen of a pregnant woman.

MENSTRUATION

In most cases, you should massage the abdomen during menstruation as it is essential for complete energy balancing. Some women prefer not to be touched on their abdomen – in this case, approach with sensitivity and ask for feedback. You could just try some gentle strokes instead of deep pressure.

CONTRAINDICATIONS

The following is a list of general contraindications for Thai yoga massage. Throughout this book, I have also highlighted specific contraindications along with the exercises to which they apply. If in any doubt, do not give a treatment. If someone has a condition that you feel unsure about it is advisable always to refer him or her to a family doctor or specialist medical practitioner for further advice.

⊕ Do not use the Stop the Blood exercises (*see pages 68 and 97*) if the receiver suffers from high blood pressure, heart problems such as heart murmurs or heart disease, or varicose veins.

⊕ Never press directly on bone or on the spine.

⊕ Do not touch open wounds, cuts, blisters or other skin conditions.

⊕ During a woman's period, avoid exercises that raise her legs over her head.

⊕ Avoid putting strong pressure on varicose veins. If you are working on energy lines in the leg you can continue with the massage as normal, until you reach the site of the varicose vein. Then you should apply very light pressure or gentle stroking only.

WATCH YOUR POSTURE

The most common postural mistakes are to work with bent arms, hunched back, tense shoulders and using your muscle strength to apply pressure. Working in this way is bound to leave you feeling achy, tired and drained after giving a massage. You will also be more likely to pick up the receiver's tension and negative energies that have been released during the massage.

The main postural rule to follow when giving a Thai yoga massage is to keep your back and, where possible, your arms straight and to apply pressure mainly using your body weight. If you remember to do this you should feel energized, relaxed and pain-free after giving a treatment.

It is always possible to keep a straight back. But there are a few exercises where it is not possible to keep your arms straight and others that require muscle power. These will be clearly indicated in the text for the relevant exercise.

If you are attempting to do a stretch that does need muscle power, take care to avoid straining yourself. If the person you are working on seems too heavy or if you feel a pulling sensation in your back, skip that exercise.

This is a good time to mention that no matter what size, level of flexibility, height, weight or age you – or the person you are working on – happen to be, you will always find Thai yoga massage exercises that you can use in comfort and safety.

If you are small and are working on a large person, you may find that certain stretches are too strenuous for you. In that case leave them out and replace them with others that are more suitable. Thai massage is very comprehensive, so there is an endless variety of stretches you can

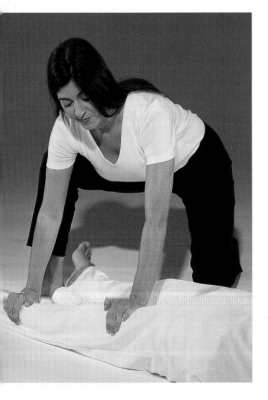

choose from – more than enough to suit everybody. We will look at planning the massage in the next chapter.

While giving the massage, keep reminding yourself of your posture and especially try to notice whether your shoulders are starting to creep up. If they are, take a breath and relax so that your shoulders go down again.

I often joke with my students that the shoulders and ears should be enemies – or at least distant acquaintances – and stay well apart. If I see a student's shoulders edging closer to their ears I tell them they are 'getting too friendly'. Keep your shoulders well away from your ears!

BODY POSITION

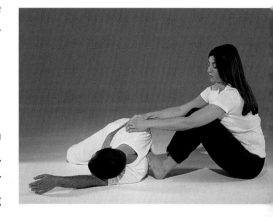

There is a difference between body posture and body position. How you hold your body is your posture, where you put your body is your position. With most of the stretches, the position that you use is either correct or incorrect and this should be clear from the text and accompanying pictures. However, sometimes it is a matter of finding a position or positions that suit you.

You may not be comfortable in the position illustrated or it may be difficult to hold for a long time. In that case you will need to be creative: there is always a way. For example, you could use cushions to kneel on or change your position more often. You should find that your comfort improves dramatically the more you practise.

The yoga exercises discussed in the last chapter are especially useful for helping you to stay comfortable in the common positions used for giving Thai yoga massage.

BE AWARE OF YOUR BREATHING

Your breathing while giving a massage is of the greatest importance. Once you become aware of your own breath you can tune into the rhythm of the receiver's breath. Being aware of your own breath is helpful for keeping you calm, concentrated and relaxed in your body. Being aware of the receiver's breath helps you to relate more deeply to them during the treatment. This, in turn, allows you to tune into the receiver's energy body and to be aware of their needs in a more intuitive way.

During the massage, try to bring your attention to your breath as often as possible. If you are getting tense or hot and bothered, simply bring your focus back to your breath and you should immediately feel calmer and more connected to the receiver.

The first time that you really become aware of the receiver's breath is during the abdominal massage. When you place your hands on their abdomen, you will feel it rise and fall as the receiver breathes in and out. Pressure is always applied on the receiver's out-breath to aid the release of muscular tension. The same principle applies to all exercises. For example, you apply the stretch on the receiver's out-breath.

In most forms of massage and bodywork, the practitioner is taught to breathe with the receiver – for example, breathing out as the receiver breathes out – whether applying pressure or a stretch. In Thai yoga massage you have a choice.

You can either use this method or you can do the opposite. In other words, while the receiver is breathing in, you are breathing out, and vice versa. This breathing method supports the energy flow but is harder to do if you are already used to the first method. Experiment with both ways to see which feels most comfortable for you.

APPLYING PRESSURE

Thai yoga massage is a strong and vigorous massage. The pressure you use should not be painful but it should be on the threshold of pain – just before it becomes painful, in other words. The amount of pressure needed to reach this level will vary from person to person. It is vital that you apply the correct amount of pressure for each individual.

This is not only important for the well-being of the receiver but also for the effectiveness of the massage. If you work too gently the massage strokes may not reach the energy body so well and thus not fulfil the purpose of the massage. If you work too strongly you may cause the receiver to feel tense and untrusting and, once again, this will not be effective.

Discovering the right amount of pressure for each person is an art in itself and takes practice and experience. At first, you will need to ask the receiver to give you plenty of feedback. When you are practising, do not hesitate to ask how the pressure feels. You would be surprised how many people will not say anything at all, even if the pressure is too strong for them, and it is even more common for people not to say that the pressure is too gentle.

It is important to mention that there are particular points or areas on the body that are usually more painful than others. These are mostly therapeutic points where it is OK to feel a degree of pain. This is what we call 'good pain'. Good pain is beneficial, as long as it is still bearable for the receiver and they can breathe and relax into it.

A good pain will disappear as soon as the pressure is released. Anyone who has had a massage in Thailand will know that if you tell the masseur that something is painful they will usually reply, 'Good for you!'

A 'bad pain', on the other hand, lasts after the pressure has been released. This indicates that the pressure was applied in the wrong point or place, or on bone.

As you practise the exercises in this book, you may come across some sore points on the receiver. Do not press too hard on these points unless you are confident that you are in the right place and are not pressing on bone. This confidence and feeling will come with time. I discuss this in more detail in later chapters.

ESTABLISHING RAPPORT

Establishing and keeping a constant connection to the receiver is vital for a good, healing massage. Even if you do not speak at all during the massage treatment, you can still develop a silent form of communication between you both that gives the receiver a sense of trust and a feeling of being cared for. This helps them to relax more deeply and let go both physically and emotionally.

Keep observing the receiver's face so that you notice any signs that might indicate that the pressure is too strong, or an area is painful, or simply that they are not comfortable with something that you are doing. Listen to the receiver's breathing and your own breathing and you may feel that they harmonize with each other as the treatment progresses.

RHYTHM AND FLOW

Another meditative aspect of Thai yoga massage is the gentle rocking movement of the giver. This constant rhythm is very relaxing and nurturing for both giver and receiver. Ideally, this rhythm should be established

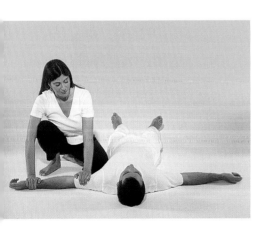

at the beginning of the massage and continue all the way through.

So often students ask me why their massage takes so long even if their rhythm is fast. I find it hard to explain, as it is to do with your ability to develop 'vision'. This means being totally present in each moment and at the same time holding a vision or intention of the next step. This difficult combination is what helps the massage to flow smoothly.

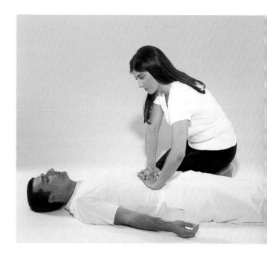

Thai yoga massage is like a painting. As you gain more experience and knowledge you have more colours to use in your painting. Sometimes, when you look at a blank canvas, you immediately have an idea of how your painting will look. At other times, you just start painting and see what develops. Likewise in Thai yoga massage. As you first touch the receiver you may or may not have a plan for your treatment but the important thing is to imagine a flow and pace that will pulse through the session.

INTIMACY AND BODY SPACE

Thai yoga massage is an intimate form of bodywork. Although the receiver is fully clothed, Thai yoga massage is often a close 'dance' between two bodies – the giver and receiver. Awareness of body space is essential to allow the receiver to relax fully and let go.

It is not uncommon for many people to have experienced some form of physical invasion or abuse in their lives. This makes it even more important to be extremely careful not to overstep physical boundaries. Always be aware of exactly where your hands are. Watch the receiver's face when you are near to sensitive areas and do not go further if you detect any sign of discomfort. Working in this way should provide the receiver with an experience of a wonderfully nourishing, safe and intimate form of non-sexual touch.

CLOTHING

Working through the clothes demands a more intuitive feeling for the body and its energy flow as you cannot rely on using your eyes to see the definition of the body. Both giver and receiver should wear loose, comfortable clothing to facilitate ease of movement. In Thailand, you will often be handed a pair of cotton trousers and a shirt to put on before your massage. I think this is a nice touch and I always have some loose cotton clothes ready in case a client turns up for a treatment in tight jeans or has come straight from the office and is wearing a suit.

The Thais are very clean people and in their warm climate it is more than likely that you will arrive for your massage with hot, sweaty feet. Therefore, often you will find that the masseur will wash your feet before the treatment. Even in a colder climate, it is not uncommon to have sweaty feet, so you may want to follow this ritual before you start the massage.

GENERAL RULES

Your fingernails should be kept short when giving Thai yoga massage. So, before you begin, always check the length of your nails and trim them as necessary. I know that for some people having short nails is a major sacrifice, but massaging with long nails is very unpleasant and painful for the receiver.

As you work through the exercises in this book, repeat each stretch two or three times. This allows the body to let go and relax a little more each time you stretch.

A good system to follow throughout the treatment is to always go to the left side first for a woman and to the right side first for a man. The reason for this is that the left side of the body is the feminine side and should be balanced first for a woman. The right is the masculine side of the body and should be balanced first for a man. Make sure that you balance the dominant side first. If you work on a woman with strong male energy, start on the right side, and if you work on a man with strong female energy, start on the left side.

However, this is not a strict rule. The most important principle is that you go to the same side first during the whole treatment. For example, when you work with one foot at a time, you go to the left foot first, then later on when you work on one arm at a time you go to the left arm first, and so on.

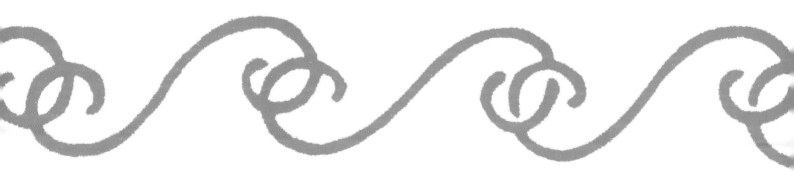

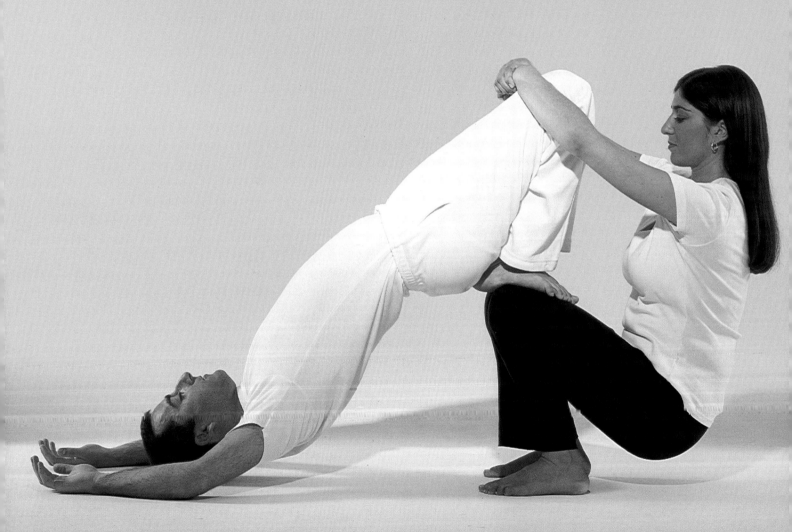

A Thai Yoga Massage Session

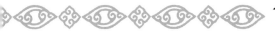

THE SESSION

It takes time and experience to build up your level of concentration. In the beginning you may well find it difficult to stay focused for very long. Therefore, when you start to practise Thai yoga massage it is best not to plan any session to last more than two-and-a-half hours. In fact, a good treatment should be between two and two-and-a-half-hours long.

Once you gain more experience, you can extend your sessions. More advanced practitioners can give a full energy balancing massage in one-and-a-half hours, but they have to cut down on the number of stretches they provide in order to do this.

I advise that you work through this chapter slowly, section by section, in the order that it is written. When you have become at ease with one part, then move on to the next. When you are familiar with the whole sequence, you can then structure the treatment you are going to give.

If you tried to include all the exercises in this book, your massage would either be too rushed or take too long. To give a complete balancing treatment it is not necessary to include every exercise, although there are certain ones that should not be left out. To help you plan your massage, I have stated which exercises are absolutely essential as I have gone along. This will be at the beginning of each new section. The others are optional, so which ones you choose should depend on the size, flexibility and needs of the receiver.

I have covered five spinal twists. It is important to include at least one of them in your massage, although there is nothing wrong with doing more than that. In the instructions for each twist I have stated who will benefit most from the exercise. You should choose the twist that is most appropriate for the receiver.

Once you are prepared, physically and mentally, to give a massage, and you have planned what you are going to do, it is time to begin. But first, it is traditional in Thai yoga massage to start with a prayer of meditation.

Meditative Prayer

One of the most important aspects of Thai yoga massage is the intention with which you give the massage. In Chapter Two we looked at some ways of preparing yourself. This includes clearing the mind, centring oneself and remembering that Thai yoga massage is the 'physical application of loving kindness'. For this reason it is very important to start your massage with a meditative prayer.

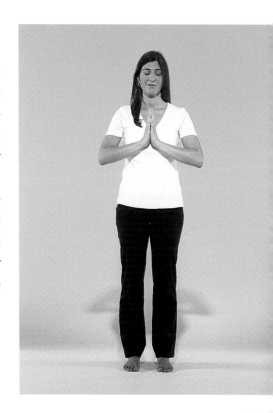

The prayer can take any form that suits you and that you feel comfortable with. It is a short way of reminding yourself of the intention behind the massage and of quietening your mind before you begin. You can stand or kneel. Simply place your hands in prayer position and close your eyes for a minute or so. In Thailand, the masseurs usually honour the founder Jivaka Kumar Bhaccha (Shivagokumarpaj).

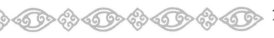 

FRONT OF THE BODY

Ask the receiver to lie on their back on the mat with their legs straight and arms by their sides. We begin the massage by loosening up the feet and ankles. This allows the receiver slowly to get used to your touch and rhythm. The rhythm and speed that you use now should be maintained throughout the massage, so try to set an easy, steady pace right from the start.

FEET AND ANKLES

STRUCTURE: You should include the basic workout on the feet in its entirety, but you can skip the second round of loosening-up exercises if you choose.

DIAGRAM 1

Therapy regions on the soles of the feet that relate to areas of the body and internal organs.

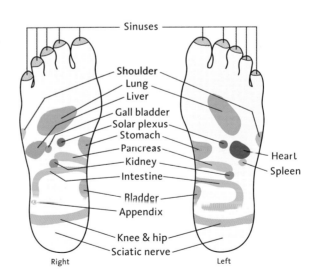

Sinuses

Shoulder
Lung
Liver
Gall bladder
Solar plexus
Stomach
Pancreas
Kidney
Intestine
Bladder
Appendix
Knee & hip
Sciatic nerve

Heart
Spleen

Right   Left

Palming the Feet

Place the receiver's feet about hip-width apart, toes pointing outwards. Put the palm of your hands on the soles of their feet, starting close to the ankles. With straight arms and back, use your body weight to press in a downwards and outwards movement. Cover the whole of the feet by moving your hands a little farther apart each time you press. This should take three to four palms, depending on the size of the receiver's feet and the size of your palms.

CAUTION: Avoid this exercise in the case of knee pain as the outward movement can put some strain on the knee.

This exercise stretches and opens up the feet, ankles and hips.

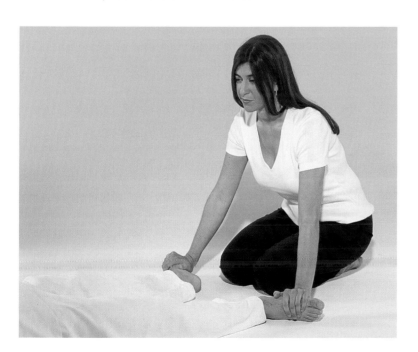

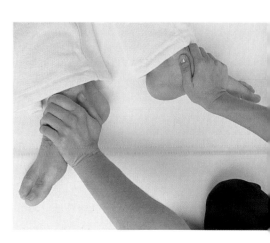

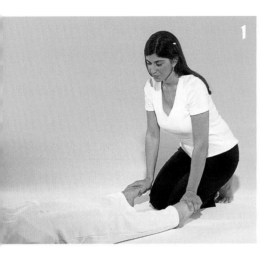

Stretching the Ankles

Place your hands on top of the feet, close to the ankles, and push straight down (1). Move your palms down the feet a little and push downwards again. Continue until you reach the toes and are pressing them towards the floor. This will be the strongest stretch on the ankles. Remember to use your body weight (2).

To stretch the ankles in the opposite direction, grasp the toes and place the heels of your hands on the balls of the feet (3). Push the feet towards the receiver's head and, at the same time, push down on the toes.

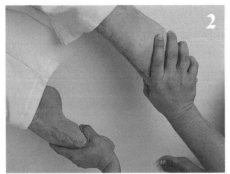

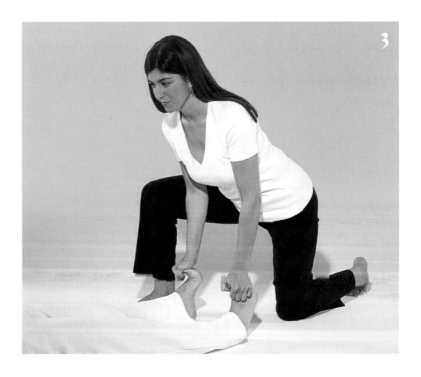

The Samosa

My students call this exercise 'The Samosa' because, in its finished position, the feet bear some resemblance to the triangular Indian pastry of that name. Holding one foot at the toes, take the foot down to the floor. Now take the other foot with your other hand and fold it on top. Place both hands on the top foot and press down. Change feet and repeat on the other side.

CAUTION: If the first foot will not go fully to the floor, do not force it but rather skip this exercise.

This exercise stretches the ankles and hips and, at the same time, puts pressure on points on the sole of the foot that tone the internal organs.

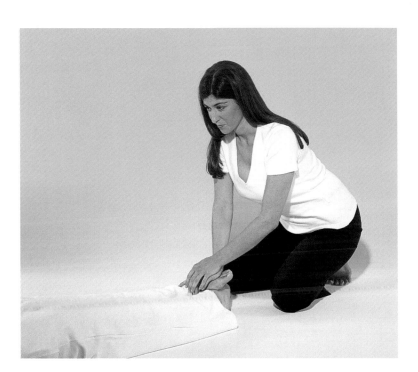

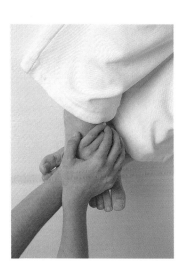

Pressure Points

If you look at diagram 1 (on page 54), you will see that wherever you press on the sole of the foot, you will be stimulating an internal organ or another part of the body. This makes covering the points on the soles of the feet extremely beneficial. There are two ways of working the pressure points on the soles of the feet.

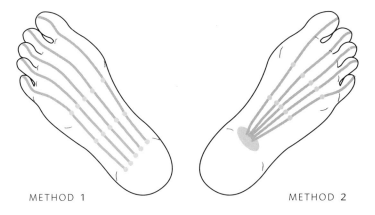

DIAGRAM 2
Therapy points on the soles of the feet that can be stimulated during a massage.

METHOD 1   METHOD 2

Method 1

Using the points for method 1 on diagram 2 as a guide, start by pressing your thumbs on the points above the heels in line with the big toes. You can do this on both feet simultaneously. Move up the feet, thumbing the points along the line until you reach the bone. Once you reach the bone, stop pressing and make rubbing movements up to the tips of the big toes. Now squeeze the tips of the toes, as this stimulates the sinuses. Repeat the same movements with each line moving up to each toe. This is the version you will use most often in a general massage.

Method 2

Using the points for method 2 on diagram 2 as a guide, start by pressing the point in the centre of the foot. It is above the heel and in line with the middle toe. This time, instead of moving straight up, follow the line in a fanning movement up towards each toe, starting at the centre point each time. In this version, you are working part of a line called *sen kalathari*. It is especially good to use this version if the receiver suffers from insomnia, heart problems or emotional tension or stress.

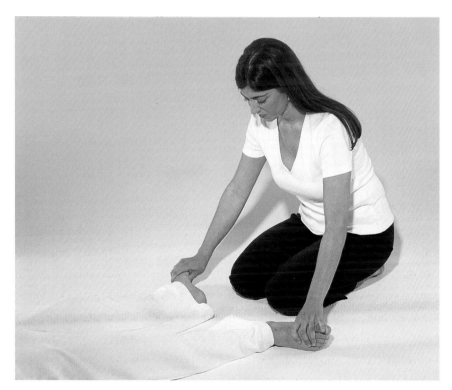

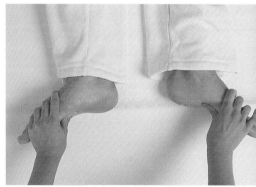

Work One Foot at a Time

Go to the left foot first if you are massaging a woman and to the right foot if you are massaging a man (*see General Rules – page 48*).

ROTATING THE ANKLE

In a kneeling position, pick up one foot. Holding it under the heel, rest the foot on your lap between your knees. With your other hand, grip the toes and rotate the foot in large circles, first clockwise then anticlockwise (1).

TWISTING THE FOOT

Hold under the heel with your inside hand. Use your other hand to grasp around the foot. Starting close to the ankle, twist the foot outwards, working your way up the foot with each movement (2). Now change hands and repeat, this time twisting the foot in the other direction (3).

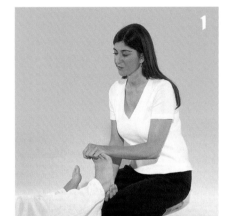

These exercises loosen and relax the ankle joints.

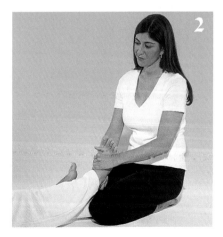

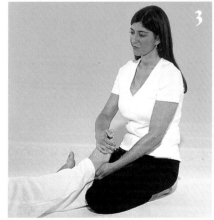

PRESSING THERAPEUTIC POINT

Now place the foot on the floor again. Press the foot back slightly towards the receiver's head. Where the foot meets the leg, you will find a depression. Place your thumb on the depression and apply pressure (1 and 2). Hold for a few seconds and release. Repeat two or three times.

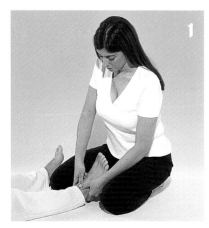

WORKING AROUND THE ANKLES.

Use fingertips to press in rotating movements all around the anklebones.

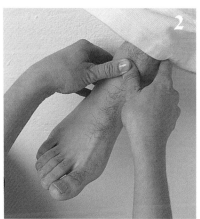

WORKING BETWEEN THE TENDONS

The *sen* lines run along the top of the feet between the tendons. Starting near the ankle, use thumb pressure to work up the foot towards the toes (3). As you are on bone here, use only gentle pressure to begin with. When you reach the soft area between the tendons, apply more pressure. Repeat until you have covered the whole area on top of the foot.

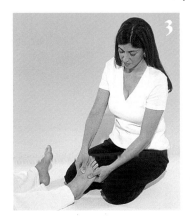

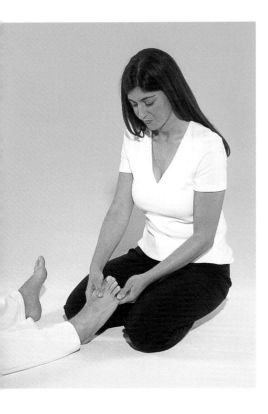

CLICKING THE TOES

Thai masseurs love clicking the joints. The more the better. In my many years of teaching I have never had a course without meeting at least one person who finds the idea and the sound of it unbearable. If that is how you feel, skip this exercise and do not force yourself to go through it. The same goes for clicking the fingers.

However, clicking the toes is perfectly harmless. In fact, for some of us it feels great. The sound that you may hear is simply caused by air trapped between the joints. I would not be representing true Thai massage if I missed it out.

Hold the sole of the foot with one hand. Use your other hand to grasp the little toe at the base, with your thumb on top. Hold firmly and pull the toe towards you and downwards with a quick, firm and confident movement. Repeat with all the toes, ending with the big toe.

CAUTION: Only click each toe once during a massage. If the toe does not make a clicking sound, do not force it or try again.

Repeat these exercises, this time using the other foot.

Now repeat all the loosening of the feet exercises, 1–5, if you wish. The feet and ankles should feel quite a bit looser now.

This exercise
relaxes the toe
joints.

Energy Lines of the Legs

STRUCTURE: Never miss out this section. This part of the massage is where you get your first real chance to work on the energy lines.

The lines do not run along precise anatomical structures, so I can give you only a general guide to their location. It is up to you to practise and use your intuition to develop a more accurate feeling for the paths these lines take. Some people have a natural, instinctive feeling for this straightaway. Others find it takes time, but this will definitely improve with experience.

We are going to work the energy lines on the legs. There are three lines running on the inside of the legs and three running on the outside. At this stage we are only going to work two of the outside lines, as the third outside line is much easier to reach later, when the receiver is lying in the side position. I have kept this workout to a minimum so it is essential to do it in its entirety. You can never do this workout too many times, so repeat it as often as you like.

Finding comfortable positions to palm and thumb the leg lines can be difficult at first. Ensure that you change position as often as necessary. Keeping a playful, rocking rhythm is also helpful.

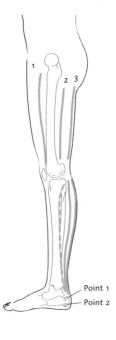

DIAGRAM 3
The energy lines
on the inside of
the leg.

DIAGRAM 4
The energy lines
on the outside of
the leg.

Inside Lines

Diagram 3

First inside line: on the lower leg, this line starts just below the anklebone and runs just under the shinbone to the knee. On the upper leg, the line starts at the inside edge of the kneecap and runs up to the groin.

Second inside line: on the lower leg, this line starts at a depression below the ankle bone located between the start of line one and line three, and runs along the middle of the calf muscle to the knee. On the upper leg, the line starts at the first obvious depression that you feel if you slide your thumb down from the inside edge of the kneecap and runs from there up to the groin.

Third inside line: On the lower leg, this line actually starts on the Achilles tendon and runs along the back of the calf to the back of the knee. On the thigh, the line starts above the tendon that you can feel there and runs up to the groin.

Outside Lines

Diagram 4

First outside line: on the lower leg, this line starts at the depression where the foot meets the leg (described in Pressing Therapeutic Point, *see page 61*), and runs alongside the shin bone up to the knee. On the upper leg, the line starts at the outside edge of the kneecap and runs up to the hip.

Second outside line: on the lower leg, this line starts at the top of the outer ankle bone and runs straight up to the side of the knee. On the upper leg, this line starts at an obvious depression that you will feel if you slide your thumb down from the outside edge of the knee and runs up to the hip.

Palming the Leg Lines

Kneel on the opposite side to the leg you are starting with. For example, if you are working on a woman, sit on her right side facing the inside of her left leg. Start by palming the inside leg. Place one hand above the ankle and the other hand above the knee. Now rock your body alternately, applying pressure from one hand to the other as you move up and down the first inside line. Now repeat this up and down the second and third inside lines. The palming should be playful and rhythmical.

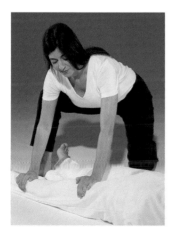
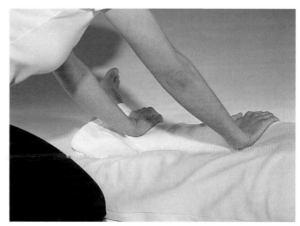

Thumbing the Leg Lines

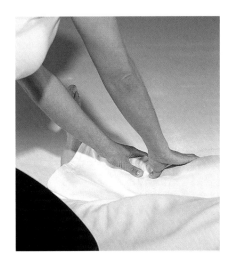

For the thumbing, work all the lines on the lower leg first and then all the lines on the upper leg. This makes it easier to find the lines and avoids moving your position too much. Start by placing your thumbs on the beginning of the first inside line. Apply pressure with the first thumb, leave a gap and apply pressure with the second thumb. As you apply pressure with the second thumb, the first thumb lifts off the line and moves into the gap. Continue walking the thumbs up and then down the line in this way.

Do the same on the second and third inside lines on the lower leg. In the same way, thumb all three lines on the upper leg. Gently rock your body from side to side as you apply pressure. Remember to keep your arms and back straight. Repeat the palming on all three inside lines.

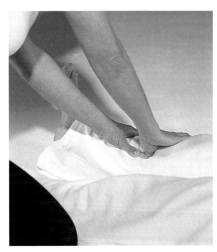

This is a good time to press the point for the sexual organs shown in Diagram 3. It is a therapy point for menstruation problems and impotence. Point 1 is located between the tip of the ankle bone and the tip of the heel. If this point is very painful, you can then press Point 2, which is directly below Point 1.

Stay where you are and work the two outside lines of the leg nearest to you. Palm the first and second lines of the outside leg. Then thumb the first and second outside lines on the lower leg, followed by the first and second lines on the upper leg. Repeat the palming.

When you have finished palming the outside lines you should add a simple stretch. Place one hand on the receiver's thigh, close to the hip, and place the other hand on the foot. Lean in with your body weight, pressing in opposite directions with each hand. Now walk around the receiver and kneel on the other side. Repeat the palming, thumbing and palming of all the lines, starting with the inside leg opposite you and then work on the outside lines of the leg nearest to you. End with the outside leg stretch.

CAUTION: When palming and thumbing the lines, do not put any pressure on or near the knees as they are very sensitive and can be very easily damaged.

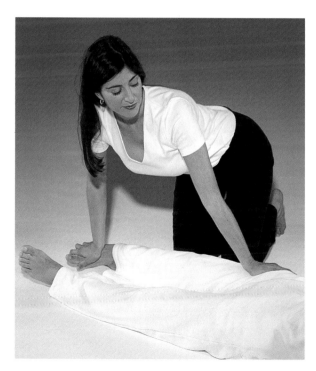

SINGLE LEG STRETCHES

STRUCTURE: You should include the Calf Stretch and Hamstring Stretch exercises coming up. Otherwise all the following stretches are optional, but try to include the Knee Across Leg Stretch as it offers a unique way to stretch the body.

This exercise cleans the blood vessels and improves circulation.

Blood Stop to the Legs

Palm up both legs at the same time until you reach the top of the leg, where you will feel the pulse. When you locate the pulse on both sides, move your hands down slightly so that you are not directly over it. Now come up on to your hands with straight arms and all your body weight. If you are in the correct place it should not be at all painful for the receiver.

Hold for about 50 seconds and then slowly release the pressure by lifting your hands. The receiver may feel a warm sensation pass down their legs as the blood flow returns.

CAUTION: Stopping the Blood is prohibited in cases of any heart condition, hypertension or varicose veins.

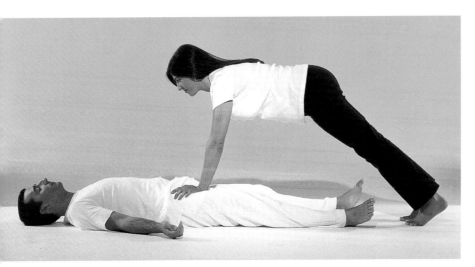

Lying Down Tree Pose

Bend one of the receiver's legs and place the foot on the floor next to the knee of their other leg. (If this is not possible, owing to stiffness in the hip, place a cushion under the bent leg.)

Palm the first inside line on the upper leg with one hand and on the lower leg with your other hand. Palm simultaneously, with both hands moving up and down the leg (1).

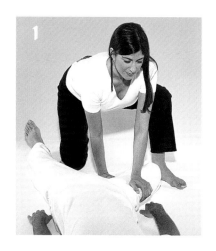

Another variation on this position is to place both palms on the thigh and simultaneously palm first and third inside lines (2).

Now place one hand on the other and palm in the middle of the thigh (3). This covers the second inside line on the thigh.

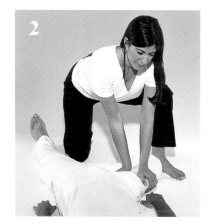

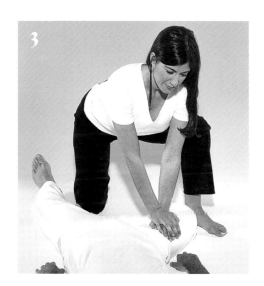

CAUTION: Do not put too much pressure on the area near the knee as it is extremely sensitive and too much pressure can cause pain.

These exercises are good for opening the hip and working the inside leg lines again.

Working the Calf

Lift the receiver's knee and place the foot on the floor. Lightly place your toes on top of the receiver's toes to stop the foot sliding. Now use your fingers to press into the middle of the calf muscle (to work the third inside line) and work your way up and down. Repeat, this time separating the muscle as you move up and down. This exercise is not only good for loosening the calf muscle it also enables you to reach the third inside line on the lower leg.

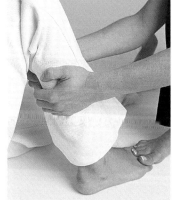

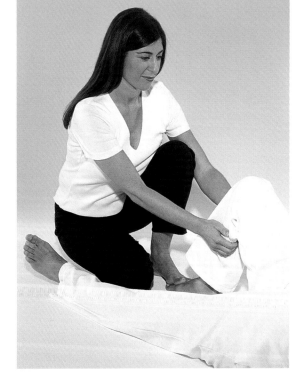

CAUTION: Do not put too much pressure on the receiver's toes.

Working the Thigh

Keeping the leg in the same position, move your body so that you are supporting the leg between your knees. Clasp your hands together and press the heels of your hands on either side of the thigh. With a slight squeezing movement, move up and then down the thigh. (This works the first inside line and first outside line.) Now open your hands a little more and move them up and down as before. (This works the second inside line and second outside line.)

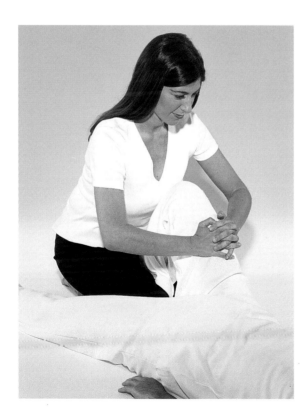

Knee Across Leg Twist

Without moving the receiver's foot, bring their knee down towards the straight leg until it rests on their thigh. Place your hand firmly on the knee so that it is held in place. With your other hand, palm up and down the whole thigh. (You can reach the first, second and third outside lines from this position.)

CAUTION: Make sure you do not put pressure on the knee of the straight leg.

This exercise works the outside lines on the upper leg again as well as providing a gentle stretch for the leg and back.

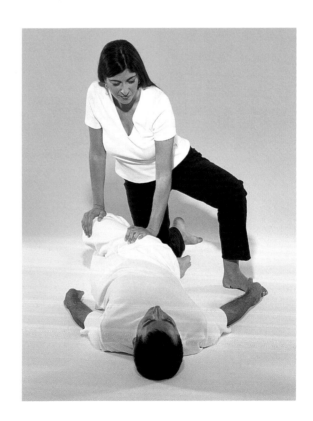

Farang Aid

In Thai, 'farang' means 'non-Asian foreigner'. This exercise is called Farang Aid because the majority of foreigners are not flexible enough to do the full pose and so need a bit of help! Kneeling, (as shown in the picture), bring the receiver's foot towards their buttocks and allow the knee to rest on your thighs. Depending on the receiver's flexibility, rest the knee higher or lower down on your thigh. If someone is very flexible you can take the knee all the way to the floor. This is no problem for most Asians. Place one hand on the knee and use the other hand to palm up and down the top of the thigh.

This exercise improves flexibility and mobility in the hip and knees.

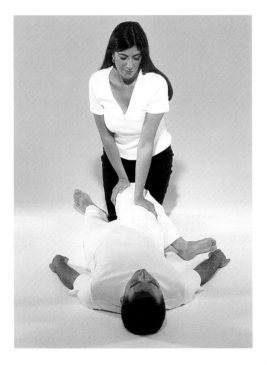

CAUTION: Always lift the knee first to bring the leg out of the position. Do not try this exercise on people who suffer pain in their knees.

Leg and Tendon Stretch

Straighten the receiver's leg and, holding the heel, take the leg out to the side until you feel resistance. Place the back of the heel over the front of your ankle. Place one hand on the knee to stabilize it. With your other hand, palm the third inside line on the thigh, just above the stretched tendon.

CAUTION: Do not work the lines on the lower leg in this position as it may put too much pressure on the knee.

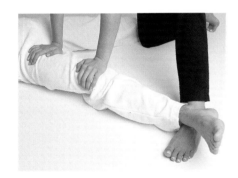

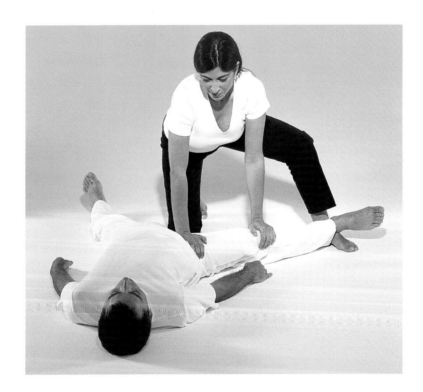

Three-way Hip Stretch

To get from the last exercise to this one, without moving your position, simply take the receiver's foot, bend the knee and place the foot on your groin area. Now adjust your leg so that you are facing the receiver straight on.

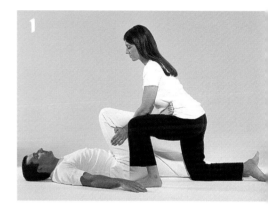

Place your hands on the back of the receiver's thigh and, using your body weight, push the leg towards the receiver's chest (1). Release the pressure and allow the leg to come up again. Move your hands a little lower on the thigh and push down again. You can repeat this a few times up and down, covering the entire back of the thigh. This is an excellent stretch for the hip and groin area. It is also effective for the relief of abdominal bloating and indigestion.

CAUTION: This exercise is contraindicated in people who have a hernia.

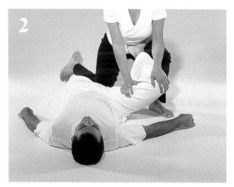

This way is similar to the previous one but, instead of pushing towards the chest, push the knee about 45 degrees away from the body. This time, use your outside hand to push on the knee and the other hand to palm the thigh (2). As before, rock in and out of the stretch each time you push. You can also hook your leg over the receiver's leg to stop it coming too far off the floor as you stretch. This stretches the hip in a second direction.

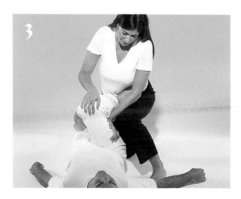

This time push the knee inwards towards the sternum (breastbone). Change hands so that your inside hand pushes the knee and your other hand is free to palm the outside lines on the thigh (3). Once again, rock in and out as you stretch. This stretches the hip in a third direction.

Paddle Boat

This exercise works the sen lines on the inner thigh and releases tension in the hamstring muscles.

From the previous position, sit back on your buttocks and place both your legs out in front of you. Allow the receiver's bent leg to fall outwards so that it is at right-angles to their torso. Place your outside foot on their thigh, behind the knee. Wrap the lower leg over your leg so that their foot goes behind your knee. Hold the heel with your outside hand. Place your other foot on the receiver's thigh and hold the straight leg with your free hand.

Now straighten your inside leg all the way. Walk your foot up and down the thigh, straightening your leg each time you have moved. As you straighten your leg, try to pull back with your body at the same time. The amount of pressure you apply in this exercise is determined by how near you sit to the receiver. The closer you are, the stronger the pressure will be. The farther back you sit, the lighter the pressure will be.

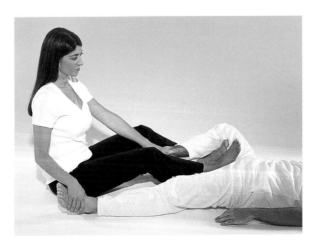

CAUTION: Avoid going too close to the groin area and do not let your foot slip.

Foot Pull

Bring the leg up so that it forms a right-angle with the body. Place your outside foot at the back of the thigh, toes pointing outwards.

Now, holding the heel and toes, pull back the receiver's foot while applying counter pressure with your foot. You can rest your other leg over the receiver's straight leg. Remember to use your body weight by leaning back as you pull.

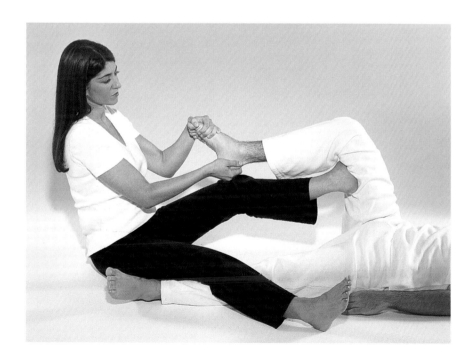

This exercise opens and gives space to the ankle and knee joints.

Thigh Squeeze

Bring the leg back into the Paddle Boat position. Place your outside foot on the middle of the thigh and bring the receiver's leg across the front of your ankle. Grasp over with your hands on to the outside of the thigh and with your fingers pull on the first and then the second outside lines. You can place both of your feet against the receiver's thigh instead, if that is more comfortable for you.

CAUTION: Pick up the calf muscle to make sure it is not pinched in this position.

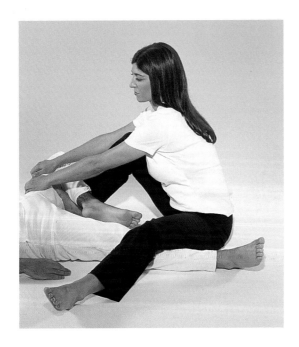
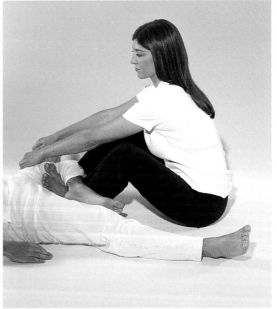

Da-dum

This exercise is made up of two movements, hence its name. Da is the first movement and dum is the second one. Generally, it is best to stand for this exercise but if you are tall and the receiver is a lot smaller than you it is also possible to kneel.

Bend the receiver's leg and, with your outside hand, push the thigh towards the sternum. With your other hand, hold the heel and push the foot in an overhead direction until there is a stretch. Try to make the movements flow smoothly into one. Repeat a few times, moving your palm up and down the thigh with each push. The straight leg may lift off the floor, but this is perfectly OK.

CAUTION: If the receiver is a woman, take care to push the thigh towards her sternum to avoid pressing on her breasts.

This exercise stretches the hamstring and hip. Palming the thigh covers the third outside line.

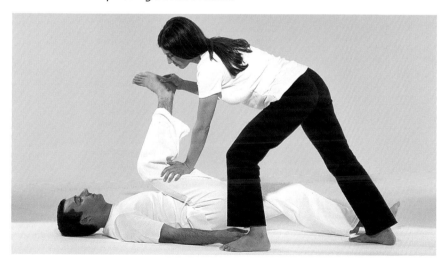

Calf Stretch

Rest on one knee with the foot of your other leg flat on the floor. Place the receiver's straight leg across your thigh. Hold the heel with your hand, forearm covering the sole of the foot. Place your other hand on the receiver's thigh. Push the top of the foot towards the shin while leaning your body forwards to support the movement. You can move your hand up and down the thigh with each stretch.

CAUTION: Avoid pressing near the knee and never apply pressure on the knee itself.

This is a great way to stretch the calf muscle.

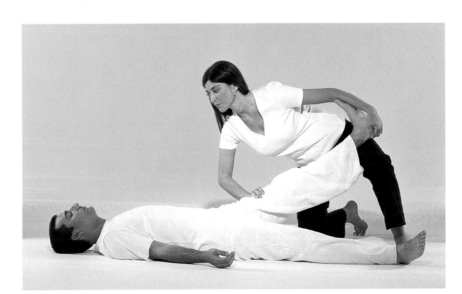

Hamstring Stretch

Kneeling down, place the receiver's straight leg on your outside shoulder. Grasp around the knee with both hands to keep the leg from bending. Bring your body up until there is a stretch (1). Release and repeat a few times. If the receiver is flexible and does not feel a stretch at 90 degrees, rather than lose your balance by leaning forwards, you will need to use your outside hand to pull down on the toes (2). At the same time, you can place your foot on the other thigh to stabilize the position. If the receiver is smaller than you are, kneel instead of standing, and use your knee instead of your foot, to stabilize the opposite thigh.

CAUTION: Do not put too much pressure on the thigh with your foot if you are standing, or knee if you are kneeling. Make sure you do not over-stretch the leg. Ask for feedback from the receiver.

This exercise stretches the hamstring.

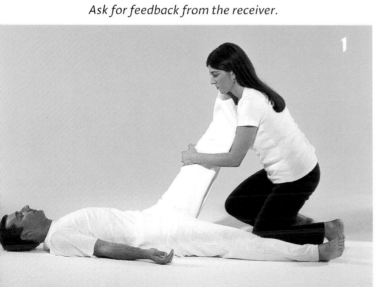

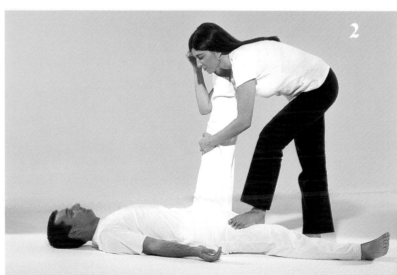

Wibbley, Wobbley

It is good to relax the leg and hips at this point, although you can do this at any time. Bend the receiver's leg and hold under the knee. Move the leg in big rotating movements, first in one direction and then the other.

Pull Over Twist

This twist is excellent for the spine and also works the back lines with the fingers.

This twists the upper part of the spine. Place the leg in Lying Down Tree Pose (*see page 69*). Sit on the opposite side and fix the leg by putting your foot on top of the bend in the leg at the knee. Take the receiver's arm and pull it over gently towards you until their shoulder comes off the ground. Reach over and work up and down their back with your fingers. This twist is ideal for flexible and fairly flexible people, but it is not good for stiff or large-bellied people.

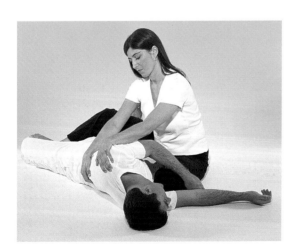

CAUTION: Do not pull with jerky movements. Make sure your knee is out of the way when you pull them over to avoid hitting their chest.

You have completed all the Single Leg Stretches on one leg. Now repeat them, this time working on the other leg.

DOUBLE LEG STRETCHES

STRUCTURE: All these stretches are optional, but try to include the Kidney Stretch. These stretches are very invigorating so they are great for people who are tired or lacking in energy.

The Plough

Lift the receiver's legs until they are at right-angles to the ground. Ask the receiver to place their hands on their knees, keeping the elbows loose, to stabilize the posture. Gently rock the legs towards the head. Start by moving only a little way and then gradually move the legs farther, depending on the receiver's flexibility. With some people, you can take their legs all the way to the floor. It is very important that the legs go straight over. If you feel them tilting to one side you can stabilize them by holding the knees yourself and asking the receiver to place their hands over their head.

CAUTION: This exercise is contraindicated in those with high blood pressure and heart disease. It is prohibited for women during menstruation as the upside down position may increase blood flow.

This exercise is good for low blood pressure. It also enhances the internal organs and aids digestion.

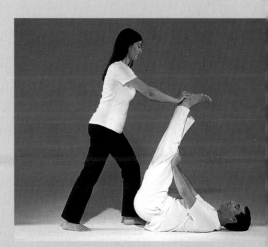

Pre-Butterfly

Ask the receiver to put their arms above their head. Step between their legs and walk up until you are standing just above the level of the armpit. Wrap their legs around your legs and bring the soles of their feet together. Hold at the ankles and slowly push their feet towards the floor.

CAUTION: This exercise is contraindicated in people with high blood pressure and heart disease and for women during menstruation. Do not force the feet all the way to the floor, as some people will find this too painful.

This exercise is good for people with low blood pressure.

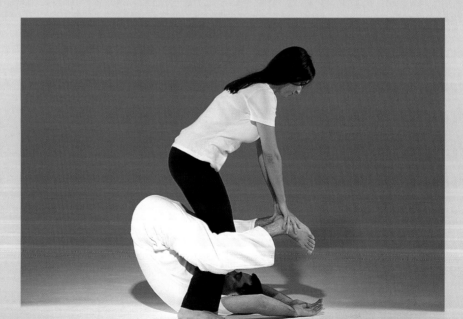

The Butterfly

Move back half a step. Wrap the receiver's legs around your legs again and bring the soles of their feet together. Push the feet straight down towards the receiver's nose. Release and repeat a few times.

CAUTION: This exercise is contraindicated in people with high blood pressure and heart disease and for women during menstruation.

This is an ideal stretch for the hips and is excellent for flexible people.

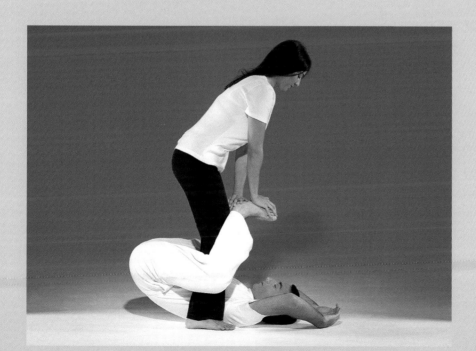

Kidney Stretch

Step back out from between the receiver's legs and bend the receiver's knees towards their chest. Place their feet against your knees. Open your feet wide and bring your knees together. Stand as close to the receiver's buttocks as possible. Lean forwards and grasp around the legs. Make sure you have a good firm grip. This exercise is easy if you do it in two parts. First, lift the receiver's knees upwards, towards your face. Second, sit back to take the knees down towards the floor. This exercise benefits the kidneys in two ways: the pressure on the feet acts on points that stimulate the kidneys and the final position stretches the kidney area.

CAUTION: Make sure you do not let go of your grip. This should avoid any problems. Do not try this on people who are much bigger or heavier than you are or who have very inflexible bodies.

This exercise benefits the kidneys.

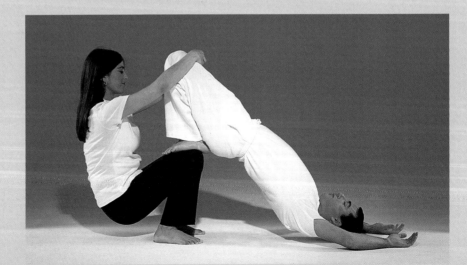

Simple Back Rest

Place your knees against the soles of the receiver's feet and lean your weight in. At the same time, push down on the shins with your hands. This is a lovely, gentle way to open and stretch out the lower back.

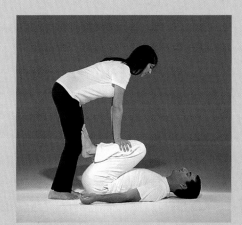

Pre-Spanish Inquisition

Straighten the receiver's legs up in the air. Bend one leg and cross the foot over the front of the other leg. Hold the ankle of the bent leg with one hand. Now palm up and down the thigh of the bent leg with your other hand. Make sure your body is towards the side so you can lean in towards the sternum. Rock forwards with your body each time you palm.

CAUTION: This exercise can be painful. Go slowly and ask for feedback.

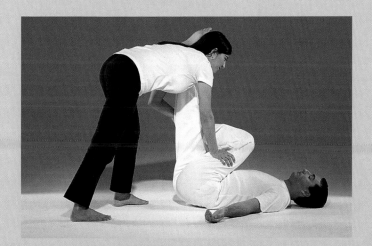

The Spanish Inquisition

This exercise is good for the lungs, digestion and kidneys.

It was Asokananda who named this exercise the Spanish Inquisition. If you have ever received it you will know why. You are unable to escape and the giver applies strong pressure to very tender points. This exercise stimulates points on the sole of the foot that relate to the lungs, digestion and kidneys. It also covers the treatment point for insomnia and emotional tension.

Keeping the receiver's legs in the same position as in the last exercise, step over the bent leg with one of your feet. Now bring the receiver's straight leg in front of your body so that it is secured and stable.

Hold underneath the foot with one hand and use the elbow of the other arm to apply pressure to points along the middle line on the sole of the foot. These points can be very painful ('good pain') but are also extremely energizing.

It is not possible to perform this on someone who is taller than you are as the foot will be too high to allow you to lean your weight in. You could try using your thumb instead of your elbow, otherwise it is best to skip this exercise.

CAUTION: There is a tendon that runs close to the points you are pressing on the side of the big toe. Be careful not to press on this tendon or slip on to it by accident.

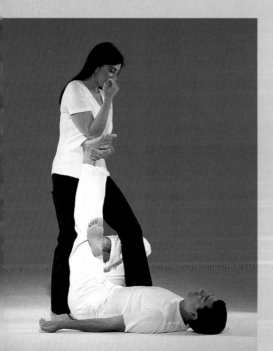

Repeat the last two exercises, this time on the other leg.

Pull Up

Straighten the receiver's legs and place them against your body. Hold the receiver's wrists and ask the receiver to hold yours. Lift the receiver by leaning your upper body back and pushing your hips forwards slightly. This brings the receiver's head towards the knees. If the receiver is taller than you are, you may not be able to do this with the legs straight up against you. In that case, open your legs a little wider, and bend your knees. Now open the receiver's legs and place them on either side of your hips.

This is a gentle exercise that benefits the spine and shoulders.

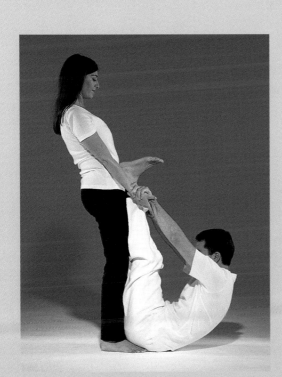

ABDOMEN, CHEST, ARMS

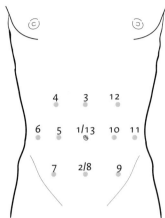

DIAGRAM 5
Acupressure points on the stomach.

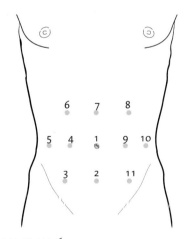

DIAGRAM 6
Acupressure points for Constipation
Variation (see page 92).

*STRUCTURE: It is essential to include an abdominal massage as all the
energy lines run through this area. Do at least one round of palming or
thumbing on the abdomen but – if possible – try to include the whole
sequence. You should include the entire sequence on the chest and arms,
other than the Blood Stop to the Arms, which is optional. Always do something on the hands. The hands are freestyle and you can spend anything
from 1 minute to 10 minutes on them.*

Abdominal massage is best performed when the receiver's stomach is
empty. Wait one hour if the receiver has had a light snack, and two to
three hours if they have eaten a heavy meal. If the receiver has recently
eaten a light meal, you could leave this entire section until later and
place it at the end of the body massage sequence before you start the
face massage.

*CAUTION: It is very important when massaging the abdomen on women
to always have their knees bent. This protects the ovaries from too much
direct pressure.*

I have already mentioned the importance of the breath in Chapter Three.
But this is a good time to remind you of it. For an effective abdominal
massage, it is essential that you tune in to the receiver's breathing. On
their out-breath, sink in very slowly with the pressure on each point.
Pause at the end of the breath and wait for the receiver's in-breath to tell
you that it is time to release the pressure as he or she breathes in.

Palming the Abdomen

Diagram 5

Always begin the abdominal massage with a few gentle strokes to let the receiver get used to being touched in this area. For a general relaxing abdominal massage, start by palming over the navel (point 1) and continue, point by point, in an anticlockwise direction, following the sequence shown in diagram 5. The distance between points is the length of the receiver's thumb.

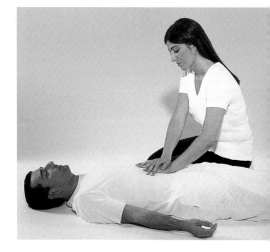

Pressing the Abdomen

This time, use the flat part of three fingers to press the points, following the same sequence as before. Be aware that by using the fingers you apply a slightly stronger, and more pointed, pressure.

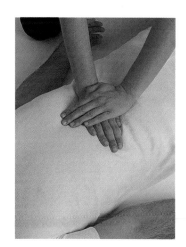

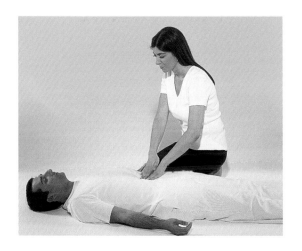

CONSTIPATION VARIATION

Diagram 6

In case of constipation it is always better to work in a clockwise direction to aid the flow of assimilation. Using your three fingers, work the points as shown in the diagram, rotating in a clockwise direction each time you apply pressure. It is important to emphasize point 11, shown on diagram 6. This indicates the end of the colon, where it is most likely to be blocked. Work this point for a longer time. It usually does wonders!

The Wave

Clasp your fingers and place your hands across the abdomen. Make wave-like movements by pushing inwards, first with one hand and then with the other.

The Scoop

Cup one of your hands inside the other. Starting at the top of the abdomen, make a scooping movement by sinking in with the side of your hands and dragging downwards at the same time. Repeat this a few times, moving down the abdomen.

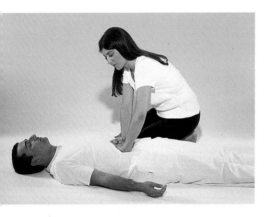

This exercise is good for pushing trapped air out of the intestines.

Thumbing Six Points

Use your thumbs to press points 4 and 1 in diagram 5.
Then points 5 and 9.
Then points 7 and 8.

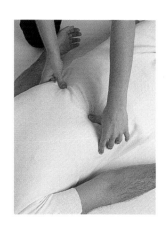

Working the Sternum

This exercise works on part of a line called *sen sumana*. It is highly beneficial for people with asthma and other respiratory problems. Place hand on hand to palm the sternum (1). Place your middle finger on the sternum and your index and ring finger on either side. Using rotating movements, work your fingers up and down the sternum (2 and 3).

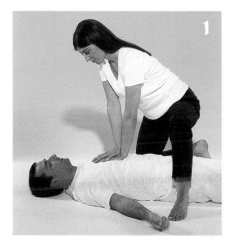

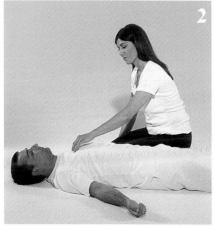

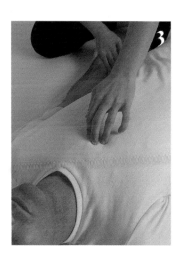

Palming Chest and Shoulders

Palm up and down the chest. Press the shoulders down by placing your palms on the soft area below the collarbone. However, if the receiver is a woman, do not press on her breasts. Simply palm below her breasts, on the rib cage, and above her breasts, at the shoulders.

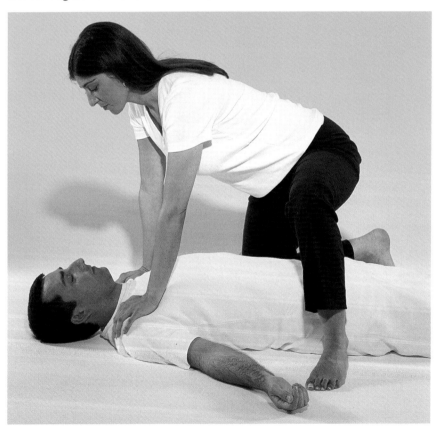

Shaking Shoulders

I also call this exercise 'Laurino's wiggle' as it was shown to me by a friend and colleague of that name. Place your fingers under the receiver's shoulders and lift them slightly off the ground. Pull alternately with your hands, playfully up and down the neck and shoulder area. Do not worry if the head moves from side to side as you do this. This is perfectly OK.

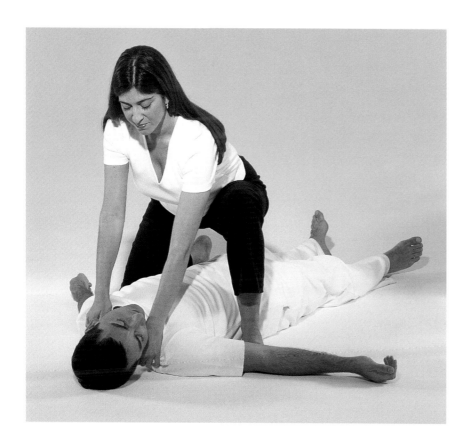

Palming and Thumbing the Arm Line

Diagram 7

We are going to cover only one main line on the inside of the arm although there are three lines in total. Do one round of palming, one round of thumbing and then another round of palming on the middle line on the inside of the arm. The lower part of the line starts at the indent in the middle of the wrist and runs straight up the middle of the forearm to the inside of the elbow. The upper part of the line runs below the biceps muscle to the armpit. When thumbing the upper arm, push upwards against the muscle instead of pressing down on to the bone, which would be painful.

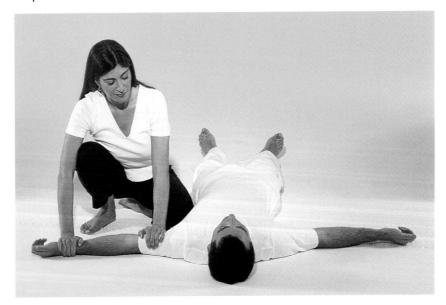

DIAGRAM 7
The main energy line on the inside of the arm.

Blood Stop to the Arm

Use one hand to grasp around the upper arm, close to the armpit. You need to almost roll the muscle up first and then press down with your body weight. You can place your other hand on top for extra weight. Apply pressure for about 30 seconds and then slowly release. If you are in the correct place, the receiver should not experience any discomfort.

CAUTION: Never do the Blood Stop with anyone suffering from heart disorders, high blood pressure or varicose veins.

Arm Pull

Place your inside foot snugly against the receiver's armpit. Hold the wrist with both hands and pull back with your body. At the same time, apply some resistance with your foot.

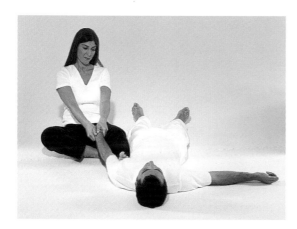

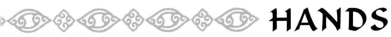

HANDS

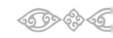

Diagram 8

Like the feet, the hands have therapy zones that relate to the whole body. Therefore, just about anywhere you press on the hands will have a beneficial effect. Diagram 8 shows some additional points used in Thai yoga massage that are useful to know.

One thing I always notice when my students are giving a hand massage is that their ears and shoulders get very 'friendly' (in other words, close together). Be aware of the position of your shoulders during the hand massage and try to find a position that allows your hand to be higher than the receiver's hand. The hand massage is mainly freestyle so you can be inventive and use your imagination. The following exercises will give you a few ideas.

DIAGRAM 8

Acupressure points on the hands.

Point 1	Hegu, relieves all kinds of pain
Points 2 + 3	For headache and toothache
Point 4	For sciatic problems and pain in the hip
Point 5	For sore throat and toothache
Point 6	For stiffness in the neck
Point 7	For pain in the shoulder and the shoulder joints
Point 8	For stiffness in the neck, pain in the shoulder and arm, stomach pain, migraine and pain in the dorsum of the hand
Point 9	For heat stroke and nausea
Point 10	For asthma, chest pain, back and shoulder pain and diseases of the wrist
Point 11	For diseases of the wrist and paralysis of the arm
Point 12	For insomnia, dream-disturbed sleep and angina pectoris
Point 13	For cough, asthma, fever, sore throat and diseases of the tendon
Point 14	For sore throat, fever, fainting and respiratory problems
Point 15	For whooping cough and arthritis of the fingers

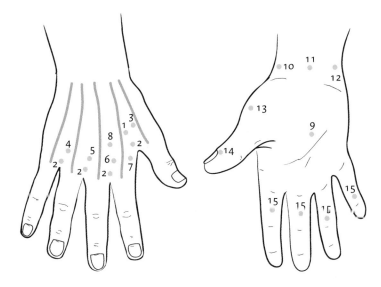

Rubbing Down Fingers

Rub down the hand, starting at the wrist and finishing at the tip of each of the fingers.

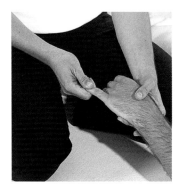

Pressing Hegu

Using your thumb, press in the soft area between the thumb and index finger, just before the bone. This point is called *hegu* by the Chinese and is also known as the 'great eliminator'. It is a very important point, as pressing it stimulates the release of painkilling chemicals called endorphins that are produced naturally in the body. Thus Pressing Hegu is an effective treatment for conditions such as headache, toothache and pain in the upper part of the body. It is also used to treat colds. Note that *hegu* is very painful when pressed.

CAUTION: This point has eliminating effects in the body and is contraindicated in pregnancy.

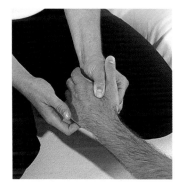

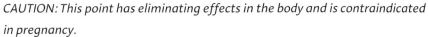

Clicking the Fingers

Grasp the receiver's little finger by placing your index finger on top and wrapping your other fingers around it. Hold firmly and make a quick, confident pull. You may hear a cracking sound. This is perfectly normal – it is only air being released from between the joints. If you do not hear a cracking sound, do not worry, simply continue with the other fingers and thumb.

CAUTION: Only try this exercise if you can do it quickly. A slow, unconfident pull does not feel good.

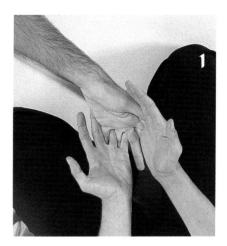 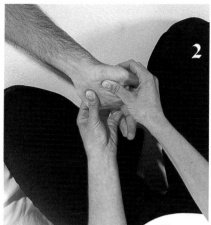

Open Palm Pressing

This is a good position in which to work the palm of the hand and it feels wonderful to receive. Turn your palms upwards and inter-link your fingers with the receiver's by placing your little fingers on either side of the receiver's middle finger (1).

Now open up the receiver's hand and use your thumbs to press on the palm. You can also stroke outwards to the fingers (2).

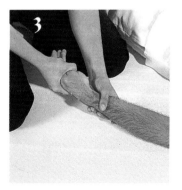

Squeezing the Hand

Hold the receiver's wrist with one hand and use your other hand to squeeze the receiver's whole hand repeatedly, moving from the wrist to the fingers (3).

Wrist Rotations

Holding the wrist with one hand, interlace your fingers with the receiver's and make circular movements to rotate the wrist in one direction and then the other.

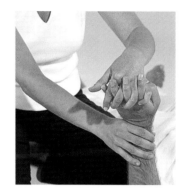

Hand Stretch

Press the fingers back with one hand and stretch the thumb back with your other hand.

CAUTION: Do not put too much pressure on the thumb as the joint is easily over-stretched.

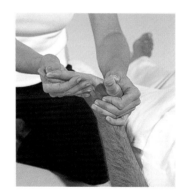

Sound of One Hand Clapping

There is an old Taoist riddle that asks, 'What is the sound of one hand clapping?' Well, I think this exercise may be the answer. Place your wrists on either side of the receiver's wrist. Alternately press up and down with each wrist, causing the receiver's hand to flap. As it touches your arms you should hear a clapping sound. This exercise is very relaxing for the wrist.

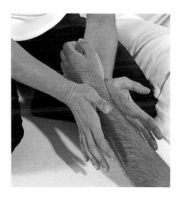

Repeat these exercises, this time working on the other arm and hand.

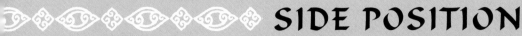 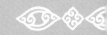

SIDE POSITION

STRUCTURE: The only essential part of this section is palming and thumbing the third outside line. But try to do a Kidney Stretch, too. Always include one of the arm stretches. If you miss them out here, you can include them in the Sitting Position section (see page 121) and vice versa.

Ask the receiver to turn on to their side. Bend their top leg and keep their bottom leg straight.

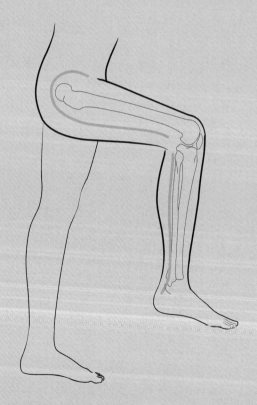

DIAGRAM 9
The third outside
energy line on
the leg.

Palming and Thumbing the Third Outside Line

Diagram 9

We have already covered three inside leg lines and two outside leg lines in the previous section. You could work on the third outside line in that section too, but it is so much easier to reach this line when the receiver is in the side position that I recommend that you work on it in this section.

On the lower leg, the line starts above the Achilles tendon and runs along the side of the tendon, next to the bone. On the upper leg, the line starts on top of the tendon at the side of the knee and runs just above the tendon. There is then an extension to the line. This extension is shaped like a boomerang and runs around the hip towards the tip of the pelvic bone. As with all leg lines, the sequence is to palm, thumb and then palm again.

CAUTION: Be aware that the 'boomerang' can be very tender.

Certain points along this line can be used very effectively for treating lower back pain and sciatica.

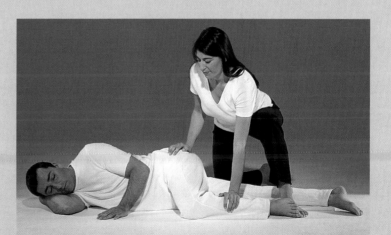

Palming and Thumbing the Top of the Arm

Place the receiver's arm, palm down, across their body. This is an easy and comfortable position for working the top of the arm. The line on top of the arm starts at the indentation in the middle of the wrist and runs up the middle of the forearm to the elbow. The other part runs up the middle of the upper arm to the shoulder. Palm the line as normal. Then thumb the line. When thumbing the upper line, at some point you will feel the bone under your thumbs. Simply skip over the bone and continue to thumb on the other side. Repeat the palming.

Gentle Arm Stretch

Place one hand on the receiver's wrist and your other hand on the shoulder. Gently push downwards and outwards with both hands.

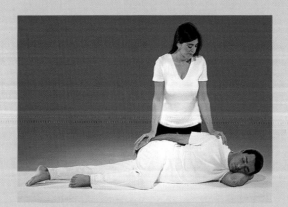

Working Behind the Shoulder-blades

Bend the receiver's arm behind their back. Use your thumbs to press in around the shoulder-blade. Place your other hand on the shoulder and pull back slightly each time you press.

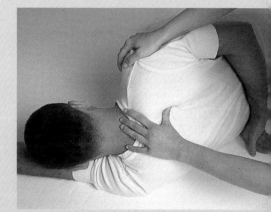

Arm Stretch

Kneel with one leg fixed against the receiver's back, just below their shoulders. Link fingers with the receiver and straighten their arm in the air. Now find the correct angle (about 45 degrees from the head) that you can stretch the arm. Move the arm in to a stretch and at the same time palm the arm, and then move out of the stretch. Repeat a few times palming up and down the lower arm and the edge of the armpit. Link fingers with your other hand and do the same thing, this time palming the other side of the lower arm and armpit.

CAUTION: You may think you are doing very little in this exercise when in fact the receiver is experiencing a very strong stretch. Always ask for feedback when doing this stretch. You will be surprised how little you have to do to make this an effective (and sometimes painful) exercise.

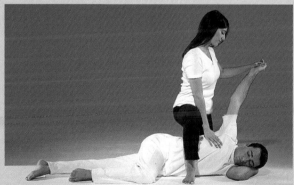

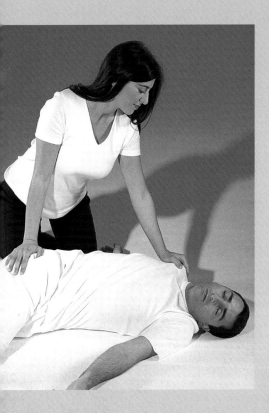

Simple Twist

This twist is good for stiff or large-bellied people. Bring the receiver's upper arm back towards the floor. Place one of your hands on the hip. Place your other hand on the soft depression next to the shoulder, under the collarbone. Keeping the hip fixed, slowly push the shoulder towards the floor. This is the most versatile of all the twists as it can be used on virtually anyone, although it is not so effective for flexible people.

CAUTION: Do not put your hand on the shoulder itself. You would then be pressing on bone and this would feel painful. Do not force the movement. Only push the shoulder down as far as is comfortable. If the receiver is very flexible you may be able to get the shoulder all the way to the floor.

Kidney Stretches

The following three exercises involve lifting and holding the receiver's leg. The leg can be quite heavy, especially if the receiver is bigger than you are. This is one of those occasions where some strength is needed. However, skip all of the kidney stretches if there is a risk that you may strain yourself.

KNEE VARIATION

Kneel behind the receiver. Pick up their top leg and hold it around the knee. Rest the leg on your arm. Place your knee in the soft area on the receiver's kidney area – between the pelvis and ribs. Use your body to lean in a curve towards the receiver's head, pulling the leg with you. When you reach a stretch, hold for a few moments and release. Repeat two or three times (1). You can also place the receiver's arm behind your back to add a shoulder stretch (2).

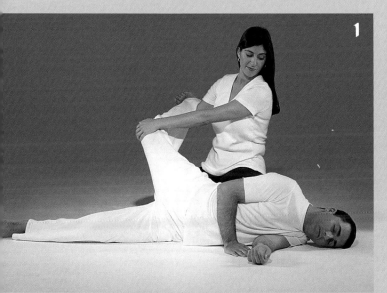
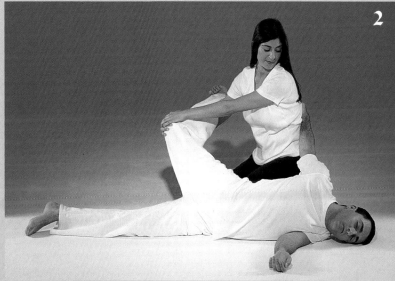

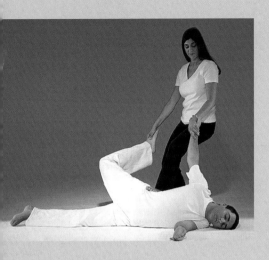

FOOT VARIATION ONE

Hold the receiver's wrist with one hand, while they hold yours. With your other hand, pick up the ankle of the top leg. Stand up, lifting the leg so that it forms a semi-circle with the receiver's body.

Now walk in a curve towards their head. At the point where you feel resistance, place your foot on their kidney area. Bend your knees to bring the receiver's leg a little lower. Then leaning back, pull their leg until there is a stretch. Repeat two or three times.

FOOT VARIATION TWO

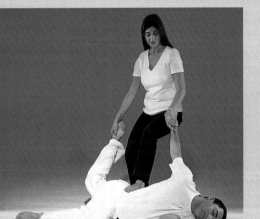

Follow the same instructions as in Foot Variation One but this time pick up the bottom leg.

In any of these three stretches, if the receiver suffers from lower back pain or weakness, you can place your knee/foot on the buttocks instead of the kidney area. It is vital that the angle of the leg is correct. You must not lift it too high or drop it too low. It is also very important that you put your knee/foot in the right place. You must avoid the ribs or pelvic bone. These exercises stretch the front of the hips and legs as well as stimulating the kidneys. They are extremely energizing.

CAUTION: Never do kidney stretches if the receiver suffers from kidney problems or has an active infection.

Lifting Twist

Stand with one foot under the receiver's bent knee. Place your other foot parallel with the first foot, against the side of the body. Cross the receiver's top arm over their bottom arm. Hold the wrist of the bottom arm while the receiver holds your wrist. Bend your knees and slowly lift the receiver by straightening your legs and leaning back with your upper body. Hold for a moment and then release. Do not use your arm muscles to pull up. If you use your body correctly, there should be no strain in this exercise.

CAUTION: Do not pull the receiver up using a jerky movement.

This twists the lower part of the spine. It is very good for flexible or fairly flexible people.

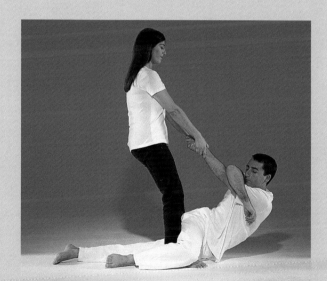

Ask the receiver to turn on to their other side. Repeat these exercises.

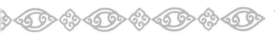 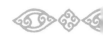

BACK OF THE BODY

STRUCTURE: Palming and thumbing the back lines is vital for a complete energy workout. Never do any less than the sequence shown. It is good to include one Cobra and make sure you include a counter-stretch to the Cobra. But the rest of the stretches in this section are optional.

Ask the receiver to turn on to their front.

Walking the Feet

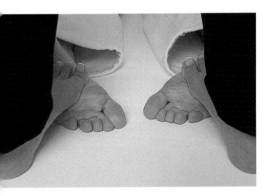

Start by placing the receiver's feet apart with the heels tilting outwards. (If the receiver finds this too difficult, leave out these exercises.) Now, walk on the receiver's instep and toes with the balls of your feet. Walk in a rocking movement by placing your weight first on one foot then on the other. For good balance, have your feet turned inwards, heels farther apart than the toes.

CAUTION: Avoid stepping on the bony area at the base of the big toe.

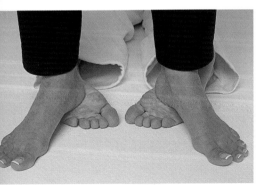

Turn around and walk on the same areas of the feet, this time using your heels. (This is slightly stronger pressure.) Keep the rocking motion but this time, for good balance, have your toes placed wider than your heels. These exercises are a wonderful way of applying pressure to some of the therapy points on the sole of the foot that tone the internal organs.

CAUTION: Again, avoid stepping on the bony area at the base of the big toe.

Stretching the Ankles

Kneel down and bend the receiver's legs by grasping the toes and pushing the feet towards the buttocks, applying pressure to the toes to stretch the ankles. Now try to stretch the ankles the other way, by placing your hands on the balls of the feet and pressing the heels towards the buttocks. You can also cross the feet by bringing the arch of one foot over the instep of the other foot and pressing down on the top foot towards the buttocks. Repeat, this time with the other foot on top.

CAUTION: Avoid doing this exercise if the receiver suffers from lower back problems. Always go slowly into the exercises and if the receiver experiences any discomfort in the lower back do not go any further.

This exercise stretches the quadriceps muscles at the front of the thighs and also releases tension in the lower back as well as stretching the ankles.

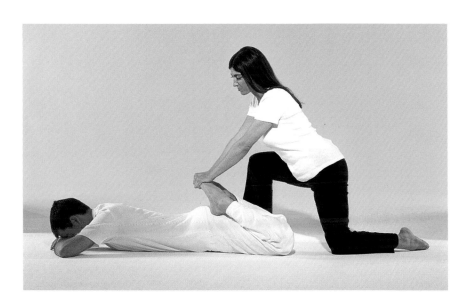

Ankle/Calf Press

Lift the receiver's feet, bend their knees, hold one foot and bring it across and down on to the other leg. Now, holding the other foot with your free hand, press the upper leg down on to the ankle-bone. You can move the lower foot up and down the leg, pressing down after each movement. Repeat, this time with the other leg on top. This exercise is good value as it uses the receiver's own body to apply pressure to the body.

CAUTION: The pressure from the ankle-bone can be very strong, so go easy.

This can be an effective exercise for relieving back pain.

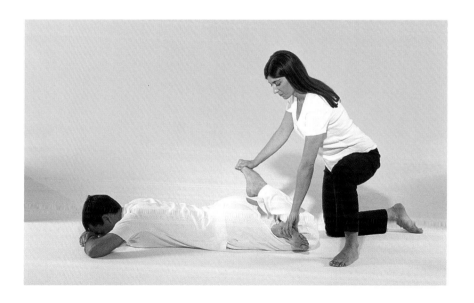

The Locust

Sit very lightly on the receiver's lower back – do not put all your weight down but just enough to stabilize the body. Place both hands around the knee of one leg, interlacing your fingers. Slowly lift the leg. As you are facing away and cannot see the receiver's face, it is important to ask the receiver to tap on the floor as soon as they feel the stretch. When you are more experienced, this may not be necessary as you will learn to feel the body's limit. Repeat with the other leg.

CAUTION: Do not do this exercise with anyone who has a weak lower back. Avoid this exercise if the person is much heavier than you are as it would be hard physical work.

This exercise stretches the front of the thigh, the hip and abdomen. It also strengthens the abdominal and pelvic muscles.

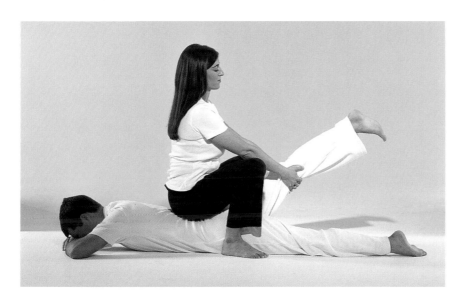

Tea Break

My students call this exercise Tea Break as it needs very little effort, giving the masseur a welcome break. If you use one hand only you could hold a cup of tea with the other hand – the receiver would never know. (I have seen this done in Thailand, but I certainly do not recommend it!) Gently lift one of the receiver's legs by the ankle and slide your legs under it until you are sitting facing outwards, close to the buttocks, with the receiver's leg over your thighs.

Placing one arm on their lower leg and your other arm on their upper leg, roll both arms outwards, away from each other, repeating the movement and moving up and down the thigh, buttocks and lower back with one arm and the calf with the other. Repeat on the other side.

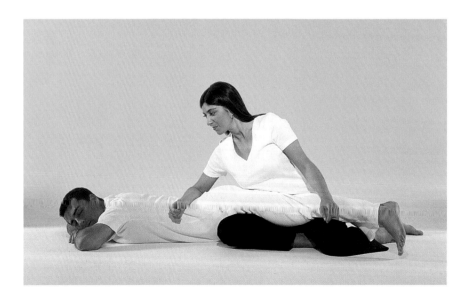

Walking the Back

Holding the foot loosely, bend the receiver's leg and step on the thigh with your weight on the arch of your foot. Move up the thigh applying pressure and then releasing. When you reach the buttocks, step over on to the back. Make sure the arch of your foot is crossing over the spine. You can now apply pressure with your foot and release as you move farther up the back.

CAUTION: Take care to apply pressure on either side of the spine but never on the spine itself. Avoid doing this exercise with anyone who is much smaller than you.

This exercise relaxes the back. It is excellent for small people who are working on larger, stockier people.

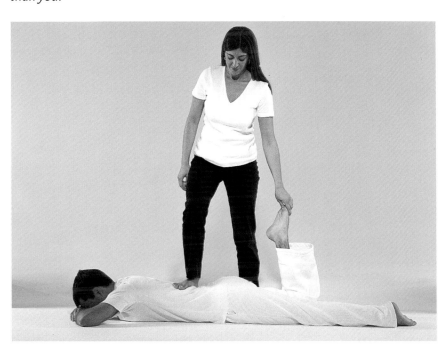

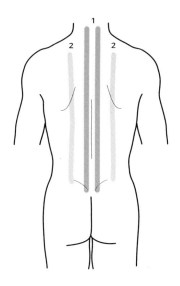

DIAGRAM 10

The energy lines on the back.

Palming and Thumbing the Back Lines

Diagram 10

Try to find a comfortable position to work the back lines. The two pictures shown here demonstrate two options. You can use one, or vary your position by switching from one to the other. If you are kneeling, it is a good idea to change sides part way through. When working the energy lines on the back, we use the same general rule as before. Start with a round of palming on each line, followed by a round of thumbing on each line, and then one round of palming again. This is the minimum workout you should do on the back lines. You can repeat it again and again.

First back line: this runs along either side of the spine.

Second back line: this runs parallel to the first back line but farther out. The distance between the two lines is equivalent to the length of the receiver's thumb.

Place your palms, fingers facing outwards, on either side of the spine. Starting at the lower back, simultaneously palm up and down the first back line. Now move your palms outwards and palm up and down the second back line. Starting at the lower back, thumb up and down the first back line and then the second back line. Repeat one round of palming along both lines.

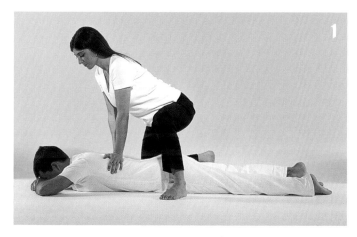

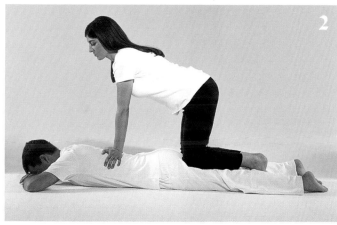

Working the Shoulders

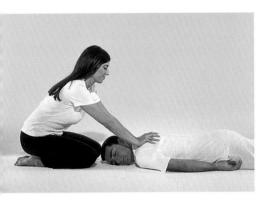

Sit above the receiver, facing the head. This is an ideal position to reach the top of the back lines. Thumb the top part of the first and second back lines. Now place your palm on the area around the shoulder-blade and make rotating movements to loosen it. Do this on one shoulder at a time. It is also effective to press the receiver's shoulders down, simultaneously, towards their feet.

Elbowing the Shoulders

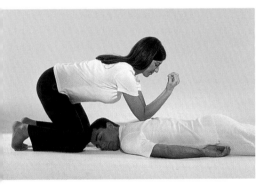

Place your elbows anywhere on the second back line and apply pressure. Work the line anywhere that you can comfortably reach. This exercise is ideal for smaller people who are working on taller or stockier people. If the receiver is much smaller than you are, skip this exercise as there will not be enough surface area for your elbows.

CAUTION: Be aware that you can apply much stronger pressure with the elbows than with the thumbs. Go easy and always ask for feedback. Avoid pressing on the spine itself.

The Cobras

These are powerful exercises that benefit the whole spine and are excellent for treating tension in the neck and shoulder. There are many variations to the basic Cobra pose. The following are the most useful ones.

COBRA ONE

This variation is for stiff, heavy people. Bend the receiver's legs up and sit on the soles of their feet. Rest the receiver's hands on your thighs above your knees. Hold the receiver around their shoulders. Slowly and smoothly, lift the receiver's body off the floor. Stay in the stretch for a few seconds and then gently lower them back down to the floor.

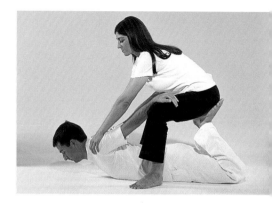

COBRA TWO

This variation is for flexible or fairly flexible people of a similar size to you. Kneel on the receiver's thighs, just below their buttocks. Hold their arms at the wrists and ask the receiver to grasp your arms. Slowly lift the receiver by pulling on the arms and leaning back as you lift them. Hold for a few seconds and then gently lower them back down to the floor.

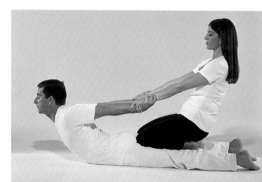

COBRA THREE

This variation works only when the receiver is bigger and heavier than you are as the receiver's weight stabilizes the position. Hold the receiver's wrists and ask them to hold your wrists. Stand on the receiver's thighs and gently pull their body up off the floor. Hold and slowly release.

CAUTION: Do not do these exercises if the receiver suffers from back problems or has any weakness in the lower back.

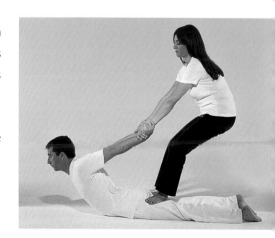

Sitting Up

Ask the receiver to turn onto their back.

Pick up the receiver's legs, allow them to bend and cross them below your knees. Holding each other's wrists, pull the receiver up. Allow the receiver to go back slowly to the floor. Repeat this twice and, the third time, once the receiver is up, walk back to bring them into a sitting position. This exercise is a clever way of bringing the receiver into a sitting position and also applies counter-stretches to the back after the Cobra.

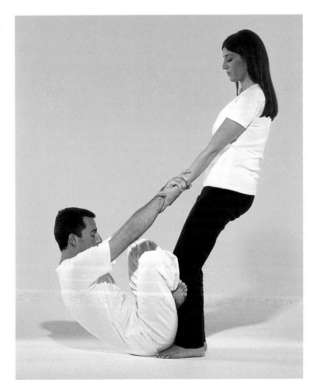

SITTING POSITION

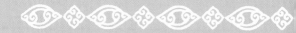

STRUCTURE: As this book is intended as an introduction to the subject of Thai yoga massage I have not put much emphasis on the shoulders and neck. Therefore it is essential that you include everything shown for those areas – palming and thumbing the points on top of the shoulders, thumbing behind the shoulder-blades, and all the work on the neck. If you have not yet included any arm stretches, you can do them now. Always include one spinal twist in the treatment.

This is another good counter-exercise for the Cobra.

Chopping

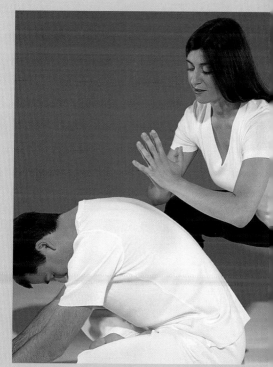

Push the receiver's body down to the floor. If the receiver is not very flexible, ask them to place their hands in front and lean their body on them instead. This is a good position for chopping. Place the palms of your hands together with fingers apart. Keeping your wrists loose, use hacking movements as you work up and down the back lines.

CAUTION: Make sure that you avoid the spine with the chopping movements.

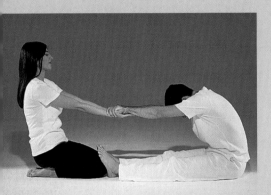

Forward Pull

Ask the receiver to straighten their legs. Sit in front and place your knees against the soles of their feet. Hold the receiver's wrists and ask them to hold yours. Lean back and pull the receiver forwards into a stretch.

Palming the Shoulders

In this exercise, you stand behind the receiver and palm the soft area on top of the shoulders. You should use different ways of palming. Start with your fingers pointing to the front, then do it with your fingers pointing to the sides, and finally with the fingers pointing backwards. Remember to lean in with your body weight as you apply pressure.

This exercise
stretches the
hamstrings and
lengthens the
lower back.
It is also a good
counter-stretch
for the Cobra.

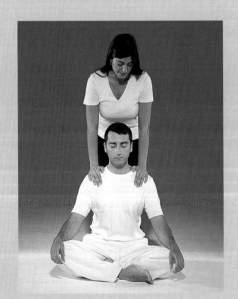

Thumbing Points on the Shoulders

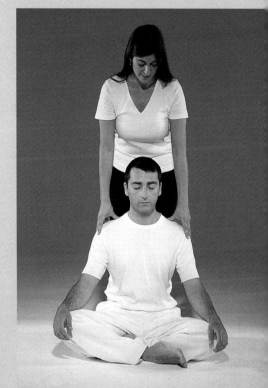

There are three important points on top of each shoulder. The first points are on either side at the base of the neck. Press them with your thumbs.

Move both hands outwards a little until you are in the middle of the muscle ridge. These are the second points. Again, press them with your thumbs.

Move outwards again until you feel the collarbone against your thumbs. Move your thumbs in a little so that you are still on the soft area and not on the bone. These are the third points. Press them with your thumbs.

CAUTION: The shoulders are common areas of extreme tension and can be very tender. Be careful when applying pressure and make sure you ask for feedback.

These exercises are
excellent for relieving
tension and stiffness
in the shoulders.

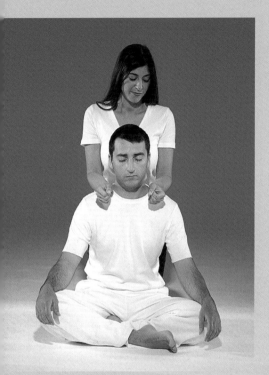

Shoulder Rolling

Kneel down behind the receiver and place your forearms on the soft area on top of their shoulders. Roll your arms outwards. Each time, move back to the same area and roll your arms again. Repeat a few times.

CAUTION: Stay only on the soft area. Do not put pressure on bone.

Neck Stretch

Use one forearm to move the head gently to one side. Clasp your hands together and place your other forearm on top of the shoulder. Press gently in an outwards movement with both arms to stretch the neck.

This is a gentle exercise to relax the shoulders.

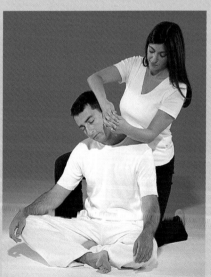

CAUTION: Take care not to over-stretch the neck. It may be difficult to judge how much to stretch. If in doubt, ask the receiver for feedback.

Neck–Elbow

Use your forearm to move the receiver's head gently to one side. Clasp your hands together and use the elbow of the other arm to press into the second point described in Thumbing Points on the Shoulders. Lean in to the elbow side only. There should be no pressure on the head.

The next four exercises are applied to one arm first and then repeated on the other arm.

This exercise stretches the neck and releases tension in the shoulder at the same time.

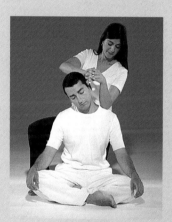

Arm Stretch

Take one arm and bend it behind the receiver's head. With your inside hand, hold the elbow and pull it towards you until there is a stretch. Use your other hand to squeeze up and down the upper arm.

CAUTION: Do not over-stretch the receiver's arm. Do not rest your arm on the receiver's head.

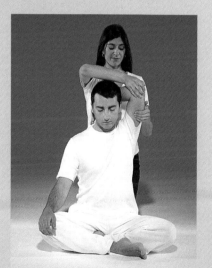

This exercise works the energy lines on the upper arm and stretches the shoulder.

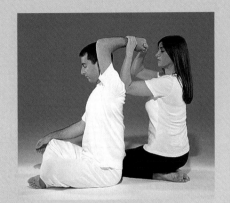

Bow and Arrow

This is one of my favourite stretches. It feels great when applied properly. Hold the receiver's wrist with your outside hand (the same side as the receiver's). Sit back on your heels. Move only your knees 45 degrees in the opposite direction to the arm you are holding. Place your elbow anywhere in the soft area between the shoulder-blade and the spine. Lean into the elbow and use your other hand to hold the fingers and pull. Between each stretch, you can move your elbow up or down to lean on different points.

CAUTION: Make sure your elbow is not pressing on the spine or shoulder-blade.

This exercise is a wonderful stretch for the arm and shoulder as well as for working points on the energy lines of the back.

Thumbing Behind the Shoulder-blades

Take the receiver's arm behind their back. Place your knee gently on the receiver's hand to stabilize the position. With one hand, grasp around the shoulder and with the other sink your thumb in to the points around the shoulder-blade. As you sink in with your thumb, you can pull back the shoulder slightly with your other hand. Go easy, as this can be a sensitive area. If you are working on a flexible person, you may be able to press your thumb right under the shoulder-blade until your thumb disappears. This exercise is great for loosening the shoulders and relieving tension.

CAUTION: Be careful not to press on bone.

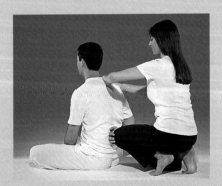

Shaking the Arm

Take the receiver's arm in front of them. Hold the hand with your two hands and give the arm a good shake. You can shake it up and down or use a circular motion.

Palming and Thumbing the Neck

Allow the receiver's head to tilt forwards. Clasp your hands and use your palms to squeeze up and down the neck. Use a pinching movement to avoid putting downward pressure on the neck. Inter-link fingers and use your thumbs to press up and down on the sides of the neck. Once again, make it a pinching movement to avoid downwards pressure on the neck.

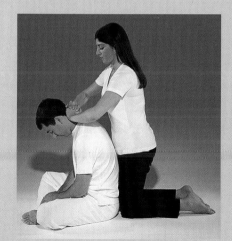 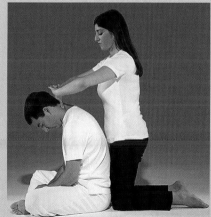

Thumbing the Head

Diagram 11

Placing thumb on thumb and starting at the base of the skull, press along the line shown all the way to the hairline. This line is good for relieving a headache and generally relaxing the head.

This line is good for relieving headaches and generally relaxing the head.

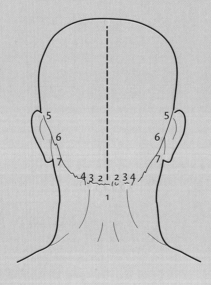

DIAGRAM 11
The therapy points on the neck and head.

Thumbing Skull Points

Support the forehead with one hand. With your other hand, thumb point 1 in the middle of the back of the neck at the base of the skull. Press your thumb upwards towards the skull. Thumb points 2, 3 and 4 on either side by moving your hands outwards slightly each time you press.

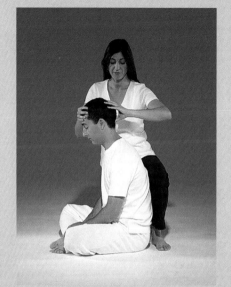

Shampooing

Use your fingers to stimulate the scalp as if shampooing the hair. As I have said before, Thai yoga massage is a complete, total massage. We do not miss out anything from the tips of the toes to the top of the head!

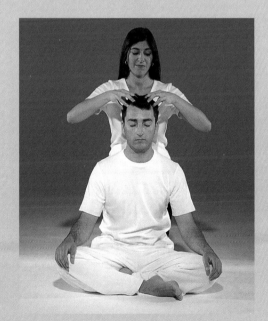

These points are very effective for relieving head and neck tension.

Smile on the Chest

Stand behind the receiver. Ask the receiver to clasp their hands behind their head. Grasp both arms, close to the armpits, and pull backwards, outwards and upwards in the same movement. Repeat, moving slightly higher up the arm each time you stretch. It is like putting a smile on the chest by opening it out.

This offers a great way to prevent drooping shoulders and sunken chest.

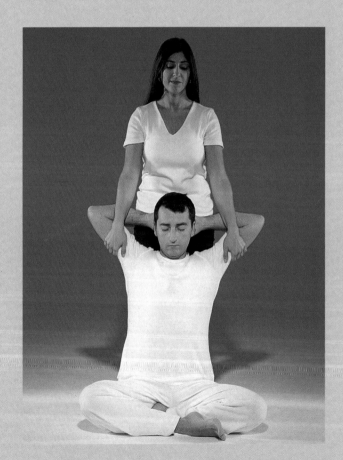

CAUTION: Take care not to over-stretch in this exercise as you cannot easily feel how strong the stretch is for the receiver.

Easy Twist

Still with the receiver's hands clasped behind their head, hold at the elbows. Stand behind the receiver with one knee and leg stabilizing their back. Place your other foot on the thigh to fix it very gently. Now turn the receiver's body by pulling the elbow that is on the opposite side to the leg that is fixed. The other hand simply stabilizes the other elbow.

This is an easy twist and is especially good for people who are not very flexible.

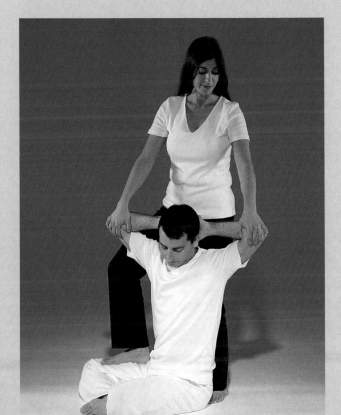

Knees in Back

Keeping the receiver's hands in the same position as in the previous exercise, place your hands between the receiver's lower and upper arms and hold near to their wrists. With your feet wide apart and your knees close together, squat down and place your knees on either side of the receiver's spine. Now press with your knees up and down the back, pulling on the receiver's arms each time you press.

CAUTION: Only press on either side of the spine with your knees. Avoid pressing on the spine itself.

This exercise works the back lines and generally loosens the back.

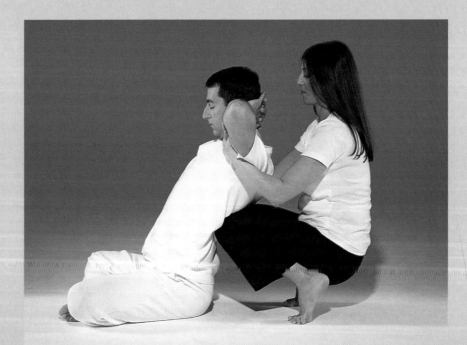

Swinging Twist

This is the king of the spinal twists as it offers the widest range of spinal movement. However, it is only good for flexible people. Bring the receiver up into a sitting position. Hold the arms as in the previous position. Fix one of the receiver's legs by placing your leg over it. Bring the receiver forwards slightly and swing their body gently until you feel that they have let you take their weight. When you feel ready, swing the receiver's torso, turning it away from the fixed leg, in one firm steady movement. Repeat on the other side.

CAUTION: This twist can only be performed with flexible or fairly flexible people. Avoid doing it if the receiver cannot let go and allow you to take their weight. Do not make any jerky movements.

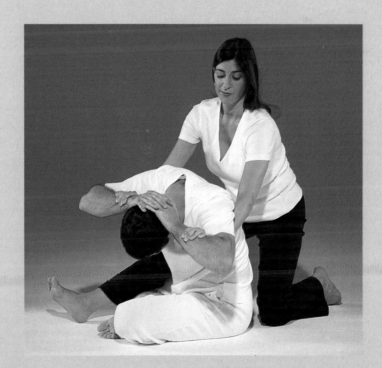

Back Walking

This exercise works the back lines with your feet and stretches the back.

Bring the receiver's arms behind their back and hold their wrists. Ask the receiver to hold your wrists. Place your feet on their back on either side of the spine, near the top. Allow the receiver's body to fall back on to your feet by softly pulling their arms. Push their body forwards again with your feet. You can then repeat the movement, moving lower down the back each time.

CAUTION: Do not walk on the spine itself. Do not pull too hard on the arms as this can cause discomfort.

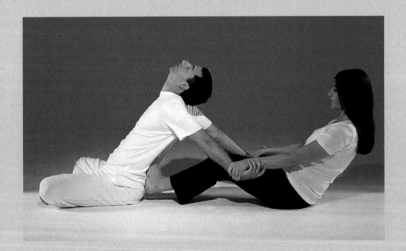

Forward Finish

Repeat Chopping and Forward Pull (*see pages 121 and 122*) to relax the back after sitting up.

THE FACE

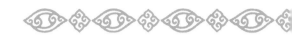

The face has many beneficial treatment points for various ailments. Always include a face massage. Like the hand massage, face massage is freestyle and you can take as little as 5 minutes or as long as 20 minutes on it. It is entirely up to you. For many people, myself included, the face massage feels like heaven on Earth! Similar to *sivasana* (Death Pose) in yoga, it allows the receiver to let go totally and relax and assimilate the massage they have received. The receiver can give up all the tension that has been released during the treatment, letting it pass into the floor.

DIAGRAM 12

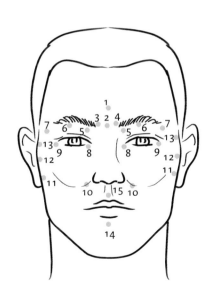

Point 1	The Third Eye – the sixth chakra
Point 2	For headache, insomnia, problems of the lower sinuses and dizziness
Points 3 + 4	For headache and facial paralysis
Point 5	For headache
Point 6	For facial paralysis and hypothermia
Point 7	For headache and facial paralysis
Point 8	For insomnia and relaxation
Point 9	For migraine
Point 10	For problems of the lower sinuses and facial paralysis
Points 11, 12 + 13	For deafness, ear pain and toothache
Point 14	For facial paralysis
Point 15	For fainting, shock, sunstroke and respiratory failure

In Thailand, the face massage can be quite rough. It is not unusual to end with a brutal chopping to the forehead. I prefer a gentler approach. As this part of the treatment is freestyle, you can really enjoy it and go with your instincts. However, there are many important therapeutic points on the face that are useful to cover. The following exercises show some of the ways to cover the facial points. It is your choice which ones you use but make sure you direct all your strokes towards the temples, as this is the most harmonious way for the receiver.

Ask the receiver to lie down.

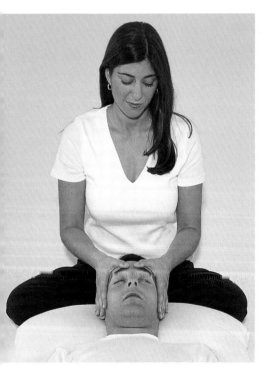

Smoothing the Frown

Starting at the centre of their forehead, between the eyebrows, stroke your thumbs outwards towards their temples, as if you are smoothing out a frown on the forehead. You can cover the whole forehead this way, starting a little higher each time.

Pinching Headache Points

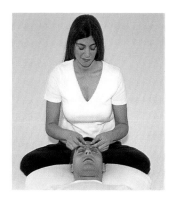

Diagram 12
Use your index fingers to press into the relevant points marked on the diagram (point 5). These are for relieving headache. (You will often see people rubbing these points instinctively when they have a headache.) Move along both eyebrows to the dip in each bony ridge about half way along (point 6). Press in this dip. This point is for hyperthermia.

Working the Temples

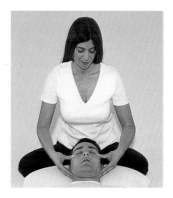

Move along to the temples and either press on them directly or use rotating movements (point 7). The temples are important treatment points for headache.

Tear Ducts

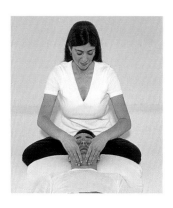

Place your thumbs on the tear ducts – the protrusions you can feel on the inside corners of the eyes (point 8). Press very lightly and hold for at least 60 seconds. These points are extremely relaxing and calming, and also very effective for treating insomnia.

CAUTION: Do not apply much pressure, as the tear ducts are very delicate. Always check whether the receiver is wearing contact lenses and, if so, do not include these points in your face treatment.

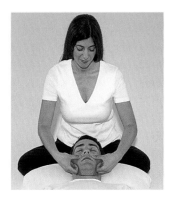

Sinus Points

Starting on either side of the nose, use your thumbs to stroke down and outwards along the cheekbones. When you reach the bottom of the nose, move outwards a little and you will find the therapy points for problems with the lower sinuses and facial paralysis (point 10).

Chin and Jaw

The sinus points are effective in the case of a blocked nose, for example as a result of a cold.

Using your thumb, press the point in the middle of the chin (point 14). This is a therapy point for facial paralysis. Now, using your fingers, make rotating movements all along the jaw line. Just before the ear you will find the area where the upper and lower jawbones meet. This area is often a source of great tension and it is advisable to spend some time relaxing it.

The Ears

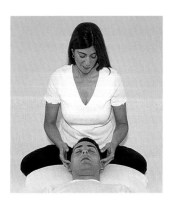

Use your index fingers to press the small depressions at the side of the ears. You will find these points where the top of the ears join the head (point 13), on the sides of the head just in front of the ears (point 12), and where the bottom of the ears join the head (point 11). These are all therapy points for deafness, tinnitus, earache and toothache. The ears themselves should not be neglected. There are 115 acupressure points on the ears that relate to the whole body. Rub the ears thoroughly all over.

Closing the Ears

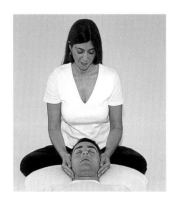

We can close our eyes to rest them but we cannot so easily give our ears a break, so it is extremely relaxing to have the ears covered for a while. (I usually find that my clients breathe a huge sigh of relief at this point in the treatment.) You have two options. You can use your thumbs to press on the protrusions at the side of the ear, or simply cup your hands over the ears. Whichever you choose, hold this position for a minute or so.

Cupping the Eyes

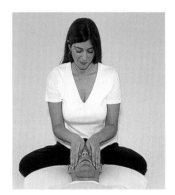

Although we can close our eyes to rest them, cupping the eyes is helpful to relax all the muscles around the eyes and is very soothing and calming. Simply cup your hands over the eyes and hold for at least a minute.

Connecting Head and Heart

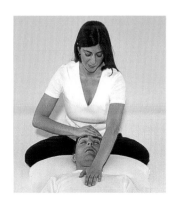

A lovely way to end the massage is by connecting the head and the heart. Place one hand across the forehead and the other over the sternum. Hold gently for a few minutes.

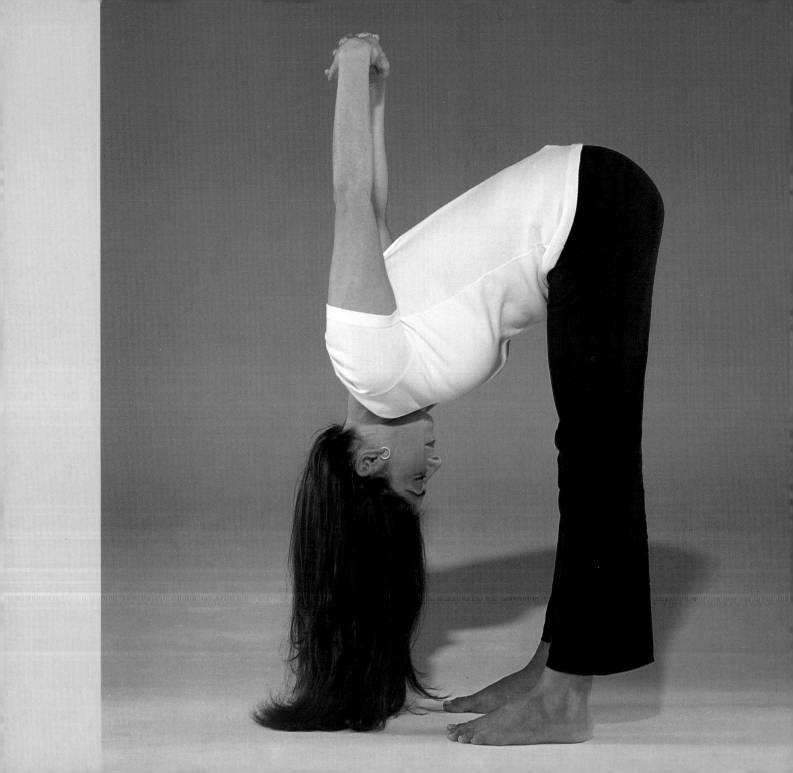

Cleansing Body
and Mind

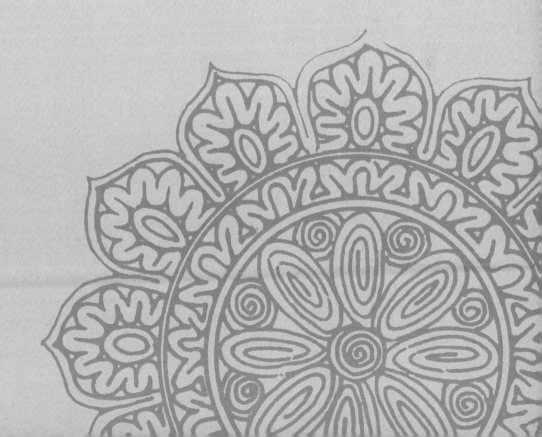

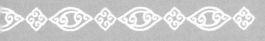

CLEAR AWAY STRESS AND TENSION

After giving a Thai yoga massage, it is essential to cleanse yourself to clear away any negative energies or stress you may have picked up from the receiver, as well as to get rid of any of your own tension that may have built up during the massage. Water is a powerful cleanser. At the very least, you should wash your hands after giving a Thai yoga massage. But when possible it is even better to take a shower.

In this chapter I have included some exercises that you can do yourself after giving a treatment, to help you relax and let go of tension. You can also use them after a hard day's work, or when you are feeling anxious or stressed.

Yoga to Rest and Release Your Back

It is amazing what a little bit of time and attention can do for your body and well-being. Simply lying on the floor for 5 minutes every day can bring immense relief to a tired back. If you can manage 10 minutes a day, then doing the simple, effective yoga routine that follows can be life-changing. I often advise my clients to spend 5 to 10 minutes a day doing these exercises. Many of them come back the following week reporting a marked improvement in posture, stress levels and back pain. But it is surprising how many come back saying that they did not have the time!

RESTING THE BACK

Lie on your back with your knees up and your feet on the floor. Allow your arms to rest on the floor by your sides with your palms facing upwards. This is an ideal position to release tension in the lower back. Take a few deep breaths and, as you exhale, imagine that an area at the back of your waist is sinking into the floor.

It is at the end of the exhalation that the body truly lets go. See if you can feel this sensation. As you breathe out, feel your shoulders drop away from your ears towards the floor. Feel the muscles at the side of your neck softening and relaxing. Let go of any tension in your jaw and face. This relaxation gives the spine an opportunity to lengthen and be free and supported.

This exercise allows the hard-working muscles on either side of the spine to take a break and really relax.

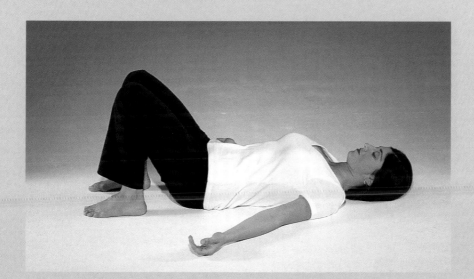

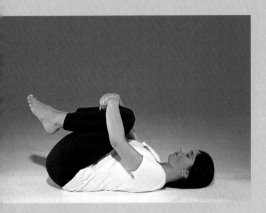

KNEES ON CHEST

Bend your knees and bring them up to your chest. Keeping your neck and shoulders relaxed, hold around your knees. To quote my mother, Mina Semyon, who is a yoga teacher, 'Holding without holding on.' In this position, the lower back is even more open. Breathe and again feel the lower back sink into the floor.

TWIST

With your knees still bent to the chest, turn your head to the left. Take your knees to the right and rest them on the floor. If you wish, you can place your hand on your top leg for support. Take a few breaths and allow your shoulder to drop towards the floor. Bring your head and then your knees back to the centre. Repeat on the other side.

This is a spinal rotation, which is very healthy for the spine as it stimulates the fluid between the spinal discs.

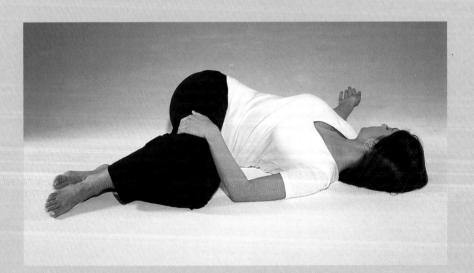

CHILD POSE

Get into a kneeling position and sit on your heels. Slowly bend forwards,
stretching your hands out in front of you. Go only as far as feels comfortable. If you cannot go all the way down to the ground, support yourself
on your hands. Take a few breaths in this position. As you breathe in, feel
your ribs expanding. As you breathe out, feel your lower back broadening
and your buttocks sinking down towards your heels.

*This is a good way
to lengthen and
gently ease out
your spine.*

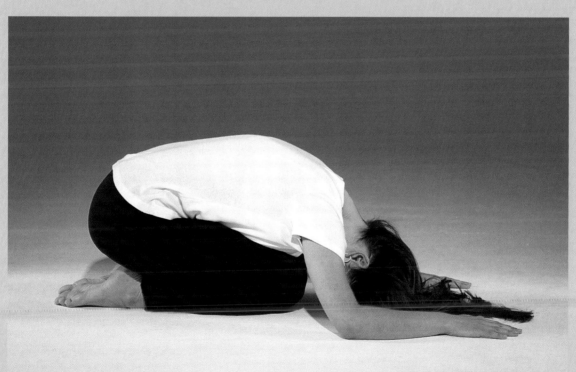

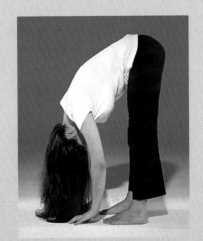

STANDING FORWARD BEND

Stand with feet hip-width apart and parallel. Slowly bend forwards from the hips; allow your upper body to hang forwards. Breathe, and really let go of your neck and head. If possible, keep your knees straight and open and avoid locking them. If you prefer, hold on to a chair as you lengthen out. You can still stretch out the spine and release the neck and head.

The Kaya Kriya

Kaya Kriya means 'body movement' and you will see why when you try it as it does involve movement of the body in order to achieve deep relaxation. The Kaya Kriya is one of the most effective exercises to use when you are left feeling drained after giving a massage or if you felt the receiver held a lot of tension or was ill. You can also use this powerful exercise when feeling stressed, low or drained of energy, or just tired.

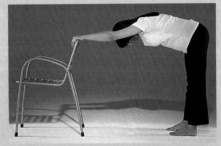

This exercise lengthens the spine and stretches the hamstrings at the back of the legs.

Although this exercise does need time, its rejuvenating effect and general benefits are definitely worth it. It is in four stages. During the first stage you focus your breath on the lower part of the lungs. During the second stage you focus on the middle part of your lungs, and during the third stage you focus on the upper part of your lungs. In the fourth and final stage you take a deep breath in and allow the air to fill all of your lungs.

To begin, lie comfortably on your back. Try to lie with your head pointing northwards to make best use of the polarity of the Earth. Place your legs comfortably apart and your arms relaxed on the floor away from your body.

STAGE ONE

Take a breath down into the lower part of your lungs and at the same time roll your feet and legs inwards as far as you can. Now, as you breathe out, roll your feet and legs outwards. Repeat 8 to 12 times.

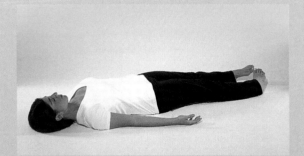 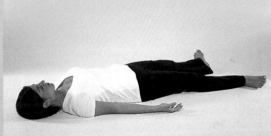

STAGE TWO

Take a breath into the middle of your lungs and at the same time roll your arms and hands outwards as far as you can. (Your back will probably lift off the floor slightly as you do this.) Now breathe out and roll your arms and hands back inwards again. Repeat 8 to 12 times.

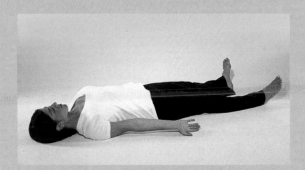 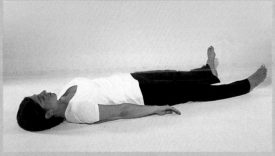

STAGE THREE

Take a breath into the upper part of your lungs and turn your head to the right. As you breathe out, turn your head to the left. Repeat 8 to 12 times.

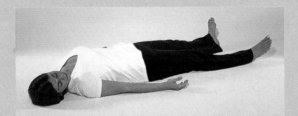 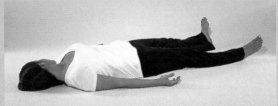

STAGE FOUR

As you breathe in, repeat all the in-breath movements you performed in the first three stages. That is, legs and feet inwards, arms and hands outwards, and head to the right. As you breathe out, do all the out-breath movements you did in the first three stages. That is, legs and feet outwards, arms and hands inwards and head to the left. Repeat 8 to 12 times. Now continue breathing normally without any effort and enjoy the relaxation position for as long as you want. The longer the better!

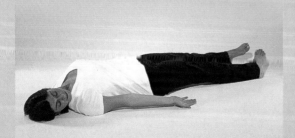 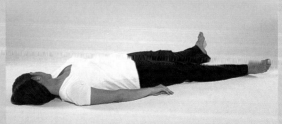

Shake Down

These are a collection of techniques that I have picked up over the years from different sources and places. I usually end my Thai yoga massage classes by doing this routine as it is a quick and effective way to cleanse, energize and centre yourself after a day of giving massage and mingling with other people's energy fields.

SHAKING THE HANDS

Stand with your feet parallel and hip-width apart. Give your hands and wrists a good shake to get rid of any tension or stagnant energy you may have picked up in your arms and hands. The shaking should be directed away from your body.

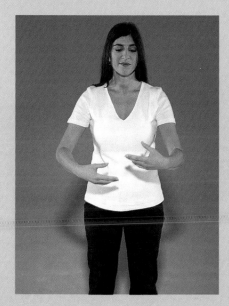 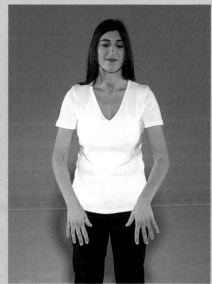

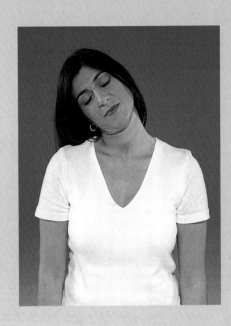

STRETCHING THE NECK

Keeping your shoulders down and relaxed, take your head to one side by bringing your ear towards your shoulder. Stop when you feel there is enough of a stretch. Hold for three or four breaths, return your head to the middle and repeat on the other side.

PUMMELLING ON THE SHOULDER

Hold your elbow with one hand for support and use your fist to pummel on your shoulder and neck area. Keep your wrists loose as you pummel. Change hands and repeat on the other side.

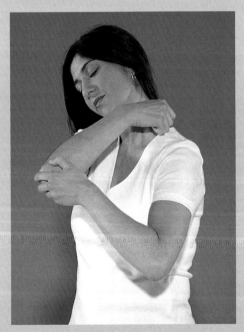

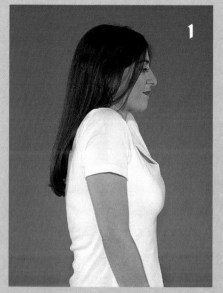
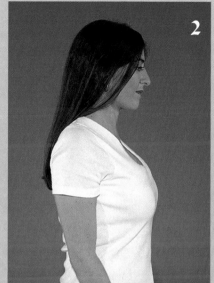
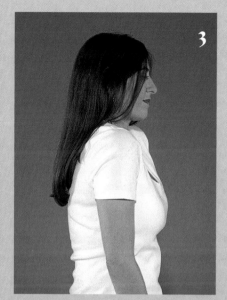

SHOULDER ROTATIONS

Slowly rotate your shoulders backwards 10 times (1–3). Now rotate your shoulders forwards 10 times.

SHOULDER SHRUG

Inhale and bring your shoulders up as far as possible towards your ears (4). Exhale and totally let go of the shoulders allowing them to drop away from the ears. Repeat 10 times.

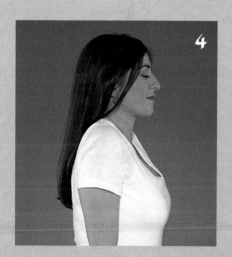

SHAMPOOING THE SCALP

Give your scalp a good 'shampooing' with the tips of your fingers. This feels very stimulating and refreshing.

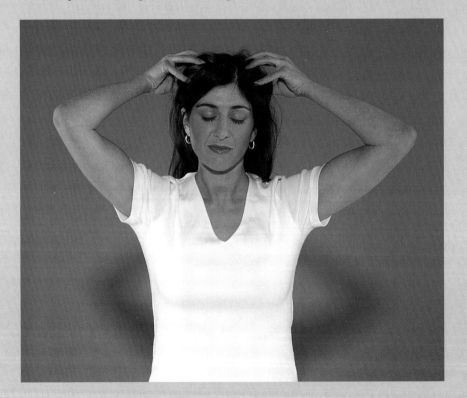

CLEANSING THE FACE

Rub your hands together vigorously and then stroke away any tension in your face using an upwards movement. Use your thumbs to smooth away any signs of a frown on your forehead.

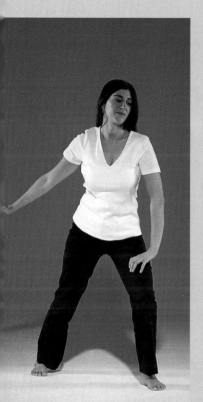
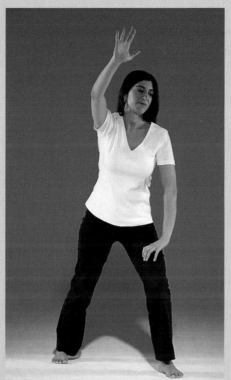
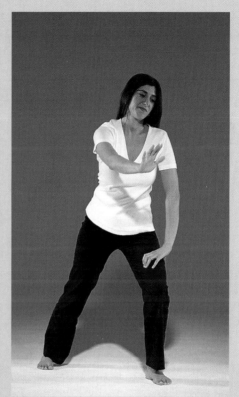

ARM SWING

Step forwards with one foot and bend the front knee slightly. Lift the hand that is on the same side as the bent leg and place it on your knee. Straighten the other arm and open the palm wide. Imagine you have a hole in the centre of your palm that is letting out all the stagnant, unwanted energy you may have picked up. Now swing your arm forwards in big circles, keeping the palm open and facing forwards. This exercise also loosens the shoulders.

RECONNECTING

Rub your hands together again vigorously and then place them one on top of the other on your *hara* – the area of your abdomen just below the navel. Close your eyes and breathe deeply. Feel the abdomen rising and falling under your hands. This area is your centre of gravity. Imagine you are connecting back to that place – that after mingling with another person's energy field you are coming back to your own energy field. As you exhale, imagine that any tension or tiredness in your body is draining out of you through your feet and heels and into the floor. As you inhale, fresh, rejuvenating energy is coming into your body and cells to refresh and replenish you.

Relaxation

This is a very simple and effective relaxation exercise for the mind and body. Lie comfortably on the floor with your arms by your sides, palms facing upwards. Place your legs slightly apart. If there is any pain or weakness in your lower back you can bend your knees and place your feet flat on the floor. Take 10 slow deep breaths to settle your body and mind.

Starting at the toes, move through every part of your body, imagining that it is relaxing. Imagine your feet, ankles, lower legs, knees and thighs relaxing. Picture your pelvis and hips letting go and sinking into the floor. Now imagine your lower back, middle back and upper back releasing tension into the floor. Relax your shoulders, arms, elbows, wrists and hands. Let the sides of the neck soften. Imagine your jaw totally letting go of tension, your eyes sinking deeper into the eye sockets and your forehead relaxing. With every out-breath, tension falls away from your body and every in-breath brings freshness and vitality into your body.

After mentally going through the whole body, take 10 more deep breaths just to relax the mind totally, then let go and do nothing.

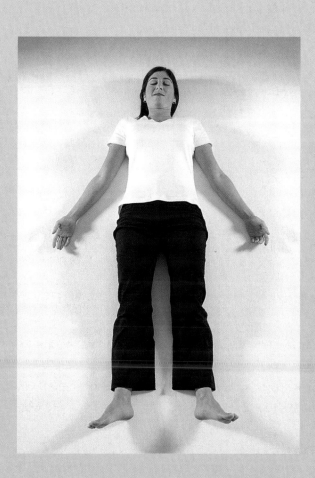

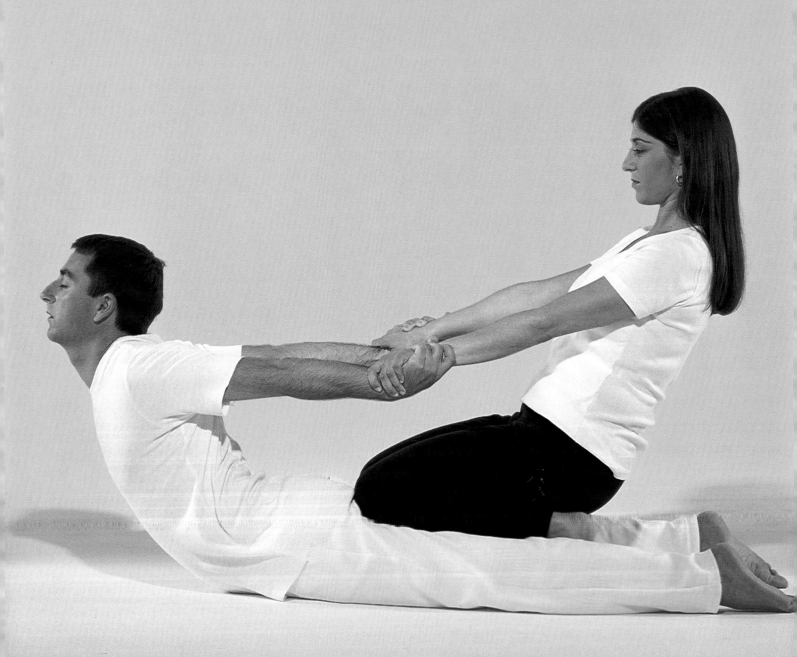

Energy and Therapy

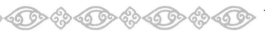

TEN SEN: ENERGY LINES

Many Eastern healing traditions are based on a system of energy lines of one form or another. All these systems differ slightly with regard to the pathways that the energy lines are said to follow. For example, the Chinese meridians differ from the Japanese meridians and the Japanese themselves follow two different systems.

All the Thai massage schools and teachers agree that there are 10 main energy lines. But they cannot agree on where the lines run. One of my teachers in northern Thailand even changes his opinions on this from year to year! Much of the written information about the *ten sen* was lost in 1767 when Burmese invaders destroyed the ancient texts. Although the epigraphs at Wat Pho remain, these only show some of the lines – not the complete line system.

Tracing the Pathways

Asokananda and his colleague, Chow Kam Thye, have carried out in-depth research over many years to come up with the following set of charts depicting the *ten sen*. This is the first work of its kind. I cannot say that these charts show the definitive paths of the energy lines, but all the hard work, experience and research that went into producing them shows that they are a genuine attempt to get as close as possible to creating a complete record of the Thai yoga massage energy line system.

I am extremely grateful to Asokananda. Thanks to his pioneering hard work, and generosity in being willing to share his knowledge with others, I am able to include these charts in this book. The most important thing to remember is that this particular energy line system does indeed work. After practising Thai yoga massage for twelve years, and being able to share in the experiences and knowledge of other practitioners, I can say this with total confidence.

These charts are useful to have as a reference. But while you are still learning the basics it is not necessary to study the charts in great detail as you will be covering all 10 lines thoroughly in the massage treatments you learn in this book.

I advise beginners simply to practise the massage. As the mechanics of the massage become more natural and easier to apply, you can then really let your intuition guide you. This is the unique freedom and beauty that you will find in the practice of Thai yoga massage as it is not weighed down by complicated theory. Thai yoga massage allows the giver to relax mentally and to rely on and develop the intuitive and feeling part of their nature.

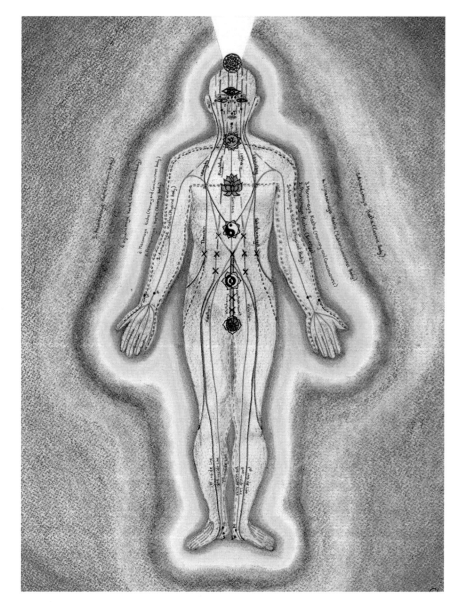

Three charts showing the ten *sen* energy lines: *Sen Sumana, Sen Ittha, Sen Pingkhala, Sen Kalathari, Sen Sahatsarangsi, Sen Thawari, Sen Lawusang, Sen Ulangka, Sen Nanthakrawat* and *Sen Kitchana.*

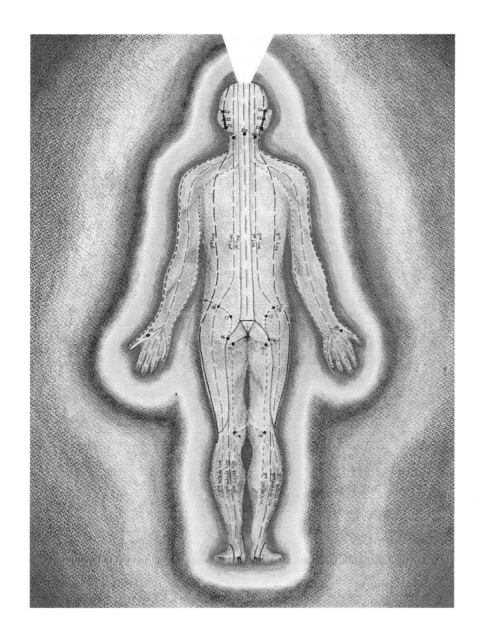

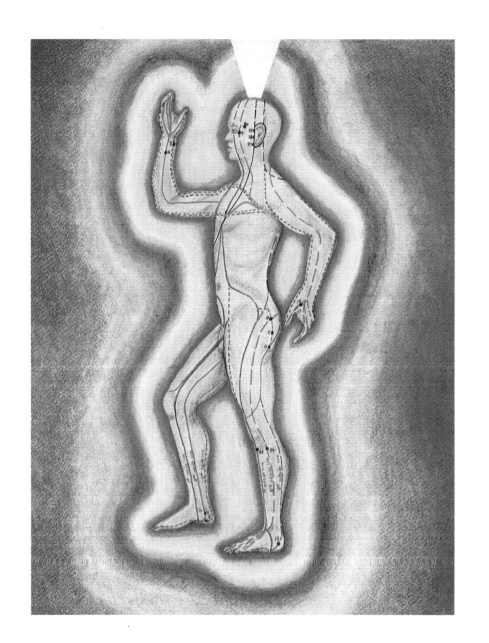

THAI YOGA MASSAGE THERAPIES

The basic massage that you learn in this book is sufficient to benefit the health and well-being of the receiver greatly. My students are always relating stories to me of the wonderful results they see during a massage session and of the feedback they are getting from delighted clients.

As you gain experience, you will develop more of an intuitive feeling for the energy body. You can then use this skill to treat specific problems and ailments. Thai yoga massage therapies cannot be standardized because they are based on the highly individual and intuitive Eastern approach. However, there are certain lines, points and stretches that have proved to be beneficial and effective for specific conditions. Therefore, keep in mind that when following these treatment guidelines there are no fixed rules. The masseur's intuitive feeling is always the most reliable and effective means of healing within the structure of Thai yoga massage.

In this chapter I have included Thai yoga massage therapy treatments for knee pain, headache and lower back pain. These are three common ailments that you are likely to come across often. We have already covered most of the energy lines, exercises and therapeutic points needed for these treatments in Chapter Four. Here it is just a matter of knowing what to include and emphasize.

APPLYING TREATMENTS

A Thai yoga massage treatment involves adding or emphasizing certain points, lines or exercises within the framework of a full body massage. As Thai yoga massage works on balancing the energy body, it is not a good idea to treat one area of the body only. The full benefit and power of Thai yoga massage comes from receiving a complete and thorough workout. The difference between providing therapy treatments and giving a general relaxing massage is that you apply much stronger pressure when working on therapeutic points. You also hold the point for longer and repeat it more often.

Always start by pressing gently, and then slowly sink in deeper and deeper. This allows the body to accept the pressure rather than resisting it. Then hold the point for 10 seconds or so. Each time you press you can increase the pressure a little more, so long as the receiver is still comfortable and able to breathe easily.

If there is too much discomfort or unease, release the pressure at once or work more lightly on that area. It is a good idea to come back to that point again and again later on during the massage. If the receiver has a problem that relates to specific therapy points, those points will usually feel more tender or may even be painful. Sensitivity on the part of the giver is needed when working therapeutically.

If a specific energy line is indicated as being beneficial for a particular treatment, you should work on it several times and come back to it as often as you like

Headache

A headache can have many causes. But this headache treatment should definitely bring noticeable relief to the receiver, whatever the cause. It may even cure some headaches completely.

FEET

Emphasize theraputic point, page 61 (1) and squeeze the tips of the toes, an area that relates to the sinuses.

ARMS AND HANDS

Thoroughly work the arm line (*see diagram 7 on page 96*) and give a full hand massage (*see pages 98–101*), thoroughly working *hegu* and the points between the fingers.

SITTING POSITION

Headaches often arise from tension in the shoulder and neck. Cover all the work on the shoulders and neck in the sitting position (*see pages 121–129*). Emphasize the points under the skull (*see diagram 11 on page 128*).

FACE

Give a long and thorough face massage (*see pages 135–139*), emphasizing all the points indicated for headache (*see diagram 12 on page 135*).

Lower Back Pain

Lower back pain can have many causes. This treatment is effective in relieving a strained lower back and for general lower back pain or discomfort. It is not intended for serious back problems such as a slipped disc.

LEG LINES

Work all the leg lines (*see pages 63–7*), emphasizing the third inside line (*see diagram 3 on page 64*).

ABDOMEN

Give a good, deep abdominal massage (*see pages 90–3*) as tension in the abdomen is often the cause of lower back pain.

SIDE POSITION

Work the third outside line on the legs (*see pages 102–3 and diagram 9 on page 102*) thoroughly, as the points around the boomerang are extremely effective in relieving back pain. Press a point behind the kneecap by placing your thumb right in the centre of this area behind the knee and applying pressure. This point is good for back pain and knee pain.

BACK OF BODY

Thoroughly work both the back lines (*see pages 116–17 and diagram 10 on page 116*). Emphasis should be placed on the first back line.

At the end of the treatment, you could also massage therapeutic oils – such as black pepper, ginger, rosemary or mayanarayan – into the back (*see Therapeutic Oils – pages 168–72*).

Knee pain

This treatment is helpful for a strained knee and can bring considerable relief to knee pain. It is by no means a cure for more serious knee injuries and problems.

FEET

Work the points on the top of the feet, between the tendons, described in Working Between the Tendons (*see page 61*). Emphasize the point described in Therapeutic Point (*see page 61*) indicated for knee pain.

LEG LINES

Work all the leg lines (*see pages 63–7*), placing emphasis on the first out-side line (*see diagram 4 on page 64*). Push the kneecap up and down with your thumbs and forefingers.

SIDE POSITION

Press the point in the middle at the back of the kneecap as used in back pain treatment.

THERAPEUTIC OILS

Aromatic massage oils, more often seen in aromatherapy, are not traditional in Thai yoga massage. However, I have found them to be a wonderful addition to the art. They are not only fragrant but also have therapeutic qualities that affect the receiver both physically and emotionally. There are two particular times when I would use oils during a massage. First, when finishing the session with a relaxing face massage and, second, after doing the line work and stretches, when they can help to relieve muscular aches and pains.

Essential oils are highly concentrated and so are extremely powerful. You must never apply them undiluted to the skin. You should combine them with a carrier oil such as almond or grape seed oil. To do this, mix about 20 to 30 drops of the essential oil with 50 ml (2 fl oz) of carrier oil. Another option is to buy good-quality massage oils ready blended.

When choosing a therapeutic oil for a massage, decide first which effect you are hoping to achieve. Do you want to relax and calm or revitalize and energize the receiver? Aromatherapy is a complex therapy and there are hundreds of oils to choose from. For now, here are a few of my favourite oils and their properties.

Energizing Oils

EUCALYPTUS

This is very stimulating and is also one of the best decongestant oils for people with colds, coughs or any other respiratory problems. Because of its energizing qualities, eucalyptus is good to use with clients who are going back to work straight after the treatment.

CAUTION: Eucalyptus oil is contraindicated in pregnancy.

LEMON

Lemon is a good reviving oil with a clean, refreshing fragrance.

ROSEMARY

Invigorating and stimulating, rosemary is said to boost circulation and relieve tired and aching muscles.

Calming Oils

SANDALWOOD

This has a meditative and peaceful quality. Sandalwood is soothing and cooling, stabilizes the circulation and the nervous system and is good for dry, chapped skin.

LAVENDER

Lavender is an excellent sedative, perfect for relaxation and treating insomnia. It is also used to relieve headaches. This oil combines well with geranium, which is a good tonic for the endocrine (hormone) system.

CHAMOMILE

Chamomile is a sedating oil, helping to ease anxiety, insomnia and stress-related headaches. It is also an excellent oil for skin disorders, such as eczema, acne and psoriasis. Chamomile combines well with lavender.

Sensual Oils

JASMINE

Jasmine has a heavenly, exotic fragrance and a sensual, pampering effect. It is one of the most expensive essences, but is extremely uplifting and luxurious. Use sparingly.

ROSE

This is another expensive oil and is very relaxing, sensual, and soothing. Rose is especially good for women pre-menstrually. Use sparingly.

CLARY SAGE

Clary sage is the ideal oil for women. It can help to relieve menstrual pains and tensions. It has a euphoric effect and can create a great sense of well-being. It is also used to treat depression and nervous exhaustion. This oil combines well with lavender.

CAUTION: Clary sage is contraindicated in pregnancy.

YLANG YLANG

This is another of my personal favourites. Ylang ylang has a very exotic floral aroma and is wonderful to use for a pampering and soothing effect. Ylang ylang combines well with sandalwood.

Oils For Muscular Relief

GINGER

Ginger is a very warming and stimulating oil. It is excellent for muscular aches and pains and very effective in relieving arthritic or inflamed joints. Ginger is also good when used in the early stages of flu.

BLACK PEPPER

This oil has a hot, stimulating effect. It dilates the blood vessels, making it very effective for the treatment of muscular aches. It is also an excellent digestive aid and is good for constipation.

MAYANARAYAN

Mayanarayan oil is not an essential oil. It is an ayurvedic oil made up of over 40 mountain herbs. It is a magical oil. It has a strong smell but is extremely effective for muscle aches, sprains and arthritic joints. Until recently, mayanarayan oil was difficult to find outside of India and Nepal. But nowadays you should be able to obtain it more easily from an ayurvedic doctor or chemist.

Resources

KIRA BALASKAS

School of Thai Massage

PO Box 33822

London

N8 8XA

Tel: 0845 0900211

E-mail: info@thaiyogamassage.co.uk

Website: www.thaiyogamassage.co.uk

ASOKANANDA

E-mail: Asokasunshine@hotmail.com

Website: asokananda.com

Information on Asokananda and the Sunshine Network in New Zealand.

Website: www.infothai.com/thaiyogamassage

Information on classes in Thailand and classes and teachers worldwide.

CHOW KAM THYE

Lotus Palm School

5870 Waverly Street

Montreal QC H2T 2Y3

Canada

Tel: (514) 2705713

E-mail: lotuspalm@hotmail.com

Website: www.lotuspalm.com

Courses in Canada and US

Bibliography

Asokananda. *The Art of Traditional Thai Massage*, Bangkok, (Harald Brust) Editions Duang Kamol 1990

Asokananda. *Thai Traditional Massage for Advanced Practitioners*, Bangkok, (Harald Brust) Editions Duang Kamol 1995

Asokananda. *Thus Have I Heard*, Bangkok, (Harald Brust) Editions Duang Kamol 1994

Maxwell-Hudson, Claire. *Aromatherapy Massage Book*, London, Dorling Kindersley, 1994

Nhat Hanh, Thich. *Peace is Every Step*, New York, Bantam Books, 1991

Tapanya, Sombat. *Traditional Thai Massage*, Editions Duang Kamol, 1990

Westwood, Christine. *Aromatherapy, A Guide for Home Use*, Dorset, Amber Publishing Ltd, 1991

Index